Natural Remedies For

Poultry

Mark Gilberd
Homoeopath. Medical Herbalist and Iridologist

Text Copyright 2012 Mark Gilberd
Global warming Edition 2024

Index

Foreword

This booklet has mainly been written for the Hobby Farmer and those who have backyard poultry; it concentrates on the diseases of poultry and gives you Herbal and Homoeopathic remedies that can be used for cure and prevention. I have mainly focused on this area and left rearing and nutrition etc alone as there are plenty of good books out there that cover these areas though there are virtually none that cover Natural Remedies for the Diseases of Poultry.

I had a very hard time trying to find all the Herbs that could be used safely for the treatment of poultry as most of this information now seems sadly lost in history. I started out with a list of the herbs that I knew poultry ate and to the list I added the herbs that I could find through history and finally added the modern herbs that are used today. After going through all this trauma I decided that I had better add a herbal to the book and make the herbs more specific to poultry so as to avoid confusion. So when you are using this book you can read up on the disease, find the herbs and go to the back of the book and find more information on the herbs you need. If any one wishes to suggest Herbs which could be added to this book safely or finds some lost in history please do not hesitate and send them to me.

The book mainly concentrates on Chickens and then goes into a little bit about Turkeys, Ducks and Geese but in reality most of these birds are attacked by the same diseases and if you find a exception just read up about the most similar you can find and adapt your treatment to that. Always try to find if you are dealing with Bacteria, Viruses, Protozoa or whatever and attack the condition using anti-bacterials, antivirals, anti- microbials in other words try to make your attack specific to the cause while trying to remove the cause at the same time.

In the Homoeopathic sections of diseases I have tried to give some of the main remedies that may suit that condition but please remember that it is said that Homoeopathy sits on a three legged stool which means that for a remedy to prove effective you need at least three strong symptoms from that remedy for a good result. In most of the write ups on disease I have included a section titled Postmortem which gives you details of what you would expect to find for a certain disease. Sometimes you have no choice but to do a Postmortem especially when your flock is dropping dead around you and you don't know what's happening. On completion of the Postmortem go on the Internet and go to The Poultry Disease Web Site as they show Postmortems for most of the diseases and here you may find your answer to what's happening. Web Address is http://poultrymed.com and it is in Israel run by a Doctor Nati Elkin. Another handy site is Merck Veterinary Manual go into Poultry then Images.

Vital Statistics

Maximum Life Span - 30 to 35 years.

Maximum Productive Life - 12 to 15 years.

Body Temperature

Adult - 103 degrees (39.5C).

Chick - 106.7 degrees (41.5C).

Respiratory Rate

Cock - 12 to 20 breaths per minute.

Hen - 20 to 36 breaths per minute.

Heart Rate

Adult - 250 to 350 beats per minute.

Chick - 350 to 450 beats per minute.

Heart rate varies with breed and sex.

Signs of Health

Comb and Wattles should be bright, full, waxy.

Eyes should be bright shiny and alert

Nostrils should be clean with no breathing sounds.

Head and Tail should be held high

Breasts should be full and plump.

Abdomen should be firm but not hard.

Posture should be erect active and alert.

Feathers should be smooth and clean.

Vent should be clean and slightly moist.

Droppings should be grey brown with white caps.

Poultry Diversification

Excellent With Chickens

Cattle, Sheep, Meat Goats - Chickens obtain nutrients from undigested feed in livestock manure and keep the flies down.

Horses - Chickens obtain nutrients from droppings and make horses less likely to spook.

Orchard - Chickens get exercise and fresh air while eliminating bugs and eating fallen fruit.

Pasture - Chickens benefit from exercise and fresh air along with green food while fertilizing the pasture

Good with Chickens

Garden - Chickens benefit from green feed and contribute fertilizer but will damage plants. You could build a Permaculture Chicken Tractor system garden.

Turkeys - Chickens gain resistance to Mareks Disease from Turkeys but also get Blackhead from them.

Poor with Chickens

Dairy Goats - Chickens foul Goat bedding and hay and the Goats eat the Chicken rations.

Pigs - Chickens and Pigs share susceptibility to Avian Tuberculosis and they may also be susceptible to a few more cross over diseases

Waterfowl - Damp conditions created by water fowl are unhealthy for chickens and ducks are very messy.

Wetlands - Damp conditions are unhealthy for chickens and water bugs transmit disease and parasites

Worms and Parasites

Usually I leave this subject alone but I will make a exception for poultry. In this Booklet Scaly Leg and Coccidiosis can be found in the Index. Worms are best treated for removal when the moon is full or on the second day of a full moon as then the worms are active and not buried in the tissues and organs.

Symptoms

Some symptoms to look for are failure to thrive, poor weight gain or weight loss, anemia, plumage especially of the wings is loose and open, eyes dull and often showing discharge, droppings often blood stained and may also be irregular ranging from constipation to diarrhea and the vent may be very soiled with faecal discharge.

Herbal Treatment

Give a course of Garlic for 10 days approximately 1 or 2 flaked cloves. Also add to the diet chopped Garlic, Onions, Wormwood, Thyme and slightly crushed pumpkin seed kernels over the days of the full moon and repeat this monthly until you are satisfied. Plenty of raw Parsley given in the diet will remedy the ravages of anemia.

For more specific information about this see Juliette de Bairacli Levys book Herbal Handbook for Farm and Stable, but the above should help you with mild infestations and keep them away after.

Respiratory System

Colds (Infectious Coryza)

This is a form of bacterial croup (Haemophilus Paragallarum) and is closely allied to the common cold of humans. The chief cause is heavy mucous accumulation usually as a result of the diet. This disease is common worldwide particularly in winter. The incubation period is 1 to 3 days.

Symptoms

Infections may be mild or severe. Eyes sticky with mucous, also mucous clogged nostrils. Breathing labored and appetite is decreased, chief symptoms are swelling of the face. Spreads mainly through contact with carrier birds. The disease can be acute and spreads rapidly or chronic and spreads slowly. Can affect chicks at least 4 weeks old and symptoms may be depression, nasal discharge, facial swelling, one or both eyes closed and death. In growing and mature birds symptoms can be watery eyes with eyelids stuck together, reddish foul smelling discharge from the nose, drop in feed and water consumption, drop in egg production, swollen face, eyes and sinuses, sometimes diarrhoea, rales or wheezing. Diagnosis is mainly through the facial swelling.

Resembles - Cholera except for the facial swelling, Newcastles Disease, Infectious Bronchitis and Influenza except for the smell of the mucous.

Postmortem Findings - Thick greyish fluid or yellowish solid material in nasal passages.

Herbal Treatment

Give Echinacea for 2 weeks so as to build up the immune system along with plenty of garlic internally, fast for one day then give a laxative diet. Latter diet should include daily Cod Liver Oil (Vitamin A) and plenty of chopped onions and mustard greens. Give inhalations of Eucalyptus oil turned into vapor in boiling water. Teaspoons of a strong Sage tea can be given. Fenugreek is a good mucous thinning herb as well as being a lymphatic cleanser and if used as a preventative it could remove the cause.

Homoeopathic Treatment

Use Potencies 6C to 30C

Aconitum - Always give at the first signs of a respiratory problem and you may stop the disease from progressing. Eyes red and inflamed with swollen lids, watering. Running nose and sneezing. There may be fever and thirst and usually there is restlessness and anxiety.

Arsenicum - Discharge is acrid, swollen eyelids with tears, chest wheezy, thirst for small quantities often, restless, irritable, worse after midnight. Dose every 2 hours for 4 doses.

Allium Cepa 6C - Discharge bland and watery, eyes red and watery and showing photophobia. Dose hourly for 4 doses.

Mercurius Sol - Much sneezing, nostrils raw with yellow greenish foul smelling discharge. Swollen eyelids with discharge.

Dulcamara - Sneezing is severe and eyes and nose are generally streaming, there can be a loose cough, the condition is usually caught from the wet and cold. Alternates well with Hepar Sulph.

Hepar Sulph 200C - Sneezing with ulceration of the nostrils, discharge thick and purulent, foul smelling, sensitive to pain, resents cold wind. Dose 3 times daily for 2 days. Is the best remedy where there has been partial relief from other remedies but not a full cure.

Laryngotracheitis

This condition is rare among free range birds. Incubation period is 6 to 8 days and the acute disease spreads slowly and may run through the flock in 2 to 6 weeks. Most birds die or recover in 2 weeks. The cause is a Herpes like virus that effects mainly Chickens and Pheasants and does not live long off the bird. The disease is highly contagious and spreads easily.

Symptoms

Congested and swollen combs of a blood red hue. Breathing is gasping and there is rattling in the throat and fluid discharge from the beak sometimes bloody.

In mild infections there may be watery inflamed eyes, swollen sinuses, nasal discharge and a drop in egg laying. In acute conditions there is nasal discharge, coughing which sometimes produces blood, head shaking, breathing through the mouth and there can be gasping, choking, gurgling or rattling sounds. A sure sign is when inhaling the fowl extends its head and neck upwards with the mouth wide open, when exhaling the head is drawn back and lowered with the mouth closed. There may be swollen sinuses or wattles, watery eyes and a drop off in egg production. This is a disease common worldwide with most of the symptoms confined to the upper respiratory tract.

Resembles - Infectious Bronchitis (bronchitis spreads more rapidly and is less severe), Newcastle's Disease but does not have nerve symptoms, Pox but there are no facial sores.

Post-mortem Findings - Swollen wind pipe clogged with bloody mucous or a cheesy plug.

Herbal Treatment

As for colds but the treatment must be immediate and more intensive. Give drops of honey as a stimulant. Give a heavy Garlic dosage and inhalations of Eucalyptus. The eyes, insides of the beaks and nostrils should all be bathed with a weak Garlic solution. Think of adding Thyme to the Sage as they both have a affinity for the throat. **Mullein** can be a good herb for this condition. Also see Chickweed.

Homoeopathic Treatment

Use Potencies 6C to 30C

Aconitum - Always give at the first signs of a respiratory problem and you may stop the disease from progressing. Eyes red and inflamed with swollen lids, watering. Running nose and sneezing. There may be fever and thirst and usually there is restlessness and anxiety.

Apis - Much edema and throat swelling, aversion to warmth of any kind and is thirstless. Give one dose three times daily for three days.

Spongia - Indicated in laryngeal conditions attended by a hoarse croupous cough, there is a absence of mucous, there may be whistling with the respiration, eyes watery, cough tends to disappear after drinking.

Drosera - Spasmodic cough associated with the upper trachea and larynx, hoarseness is very pronounced, there is also tenacious mucous, the cough usually produces reaching and vomiting and greatly impedes breathing.

Phytolacca - Useful in those cases where a membranous deposit covers the affected area, marked redness of the larynx, pain, rapid and weak pulse there is a state of restlessness and prostration, eye discharge, dry cough.

Causticum - Indicated in those cases where the voice becomes lost due to a temporary paralysis of the laryngeal nerves, mucous gathers in the throat with great difficulty expelling it, harsh dry cough, inflammation of the eyelids.

Kali Bich - Mucous of a tough stringy nature colored yellow, discharges with edema of the eyelids, catarrhal inflammation of the sinuses, papular eruptions with ulcers, worse from cold, better for heat.

Infectious Bronchitis

Can be known as chick bronchitis or Gasping Disease. This disease is fairly common and has a incubation period of 18 to 36 hours then the acute condition starts suddenly and spreads rapidly and can run through the flock in 24 to 48 hours. Individuals recover in about 2 to 3 weeks. The cause is several strains of the Coronavirus which can survive for one week off the bird and only effects chickens. The virus can be easily destroyed by disinfectants. One of the most contagious of the poultry diseases

Symptoms

In birds of all ages there may be gasping, coughing, sneezing, rattling, wet eyes and a nasal discharge. In young growing birds there may be a watery nasal discharge, huddling near heat, loss of appetite, head shaking, slow growth and sometimes swollen sinuses. In maturing birds there is sometime a swollen wattle. In hens there is a sharp drop off in laying to near zero and the eggs may be thin, soft and misshapen or rigid shells with watery whites.

Resembles - Laryngotracheitis but spreads faster and is less severe, Infectious Coryza but does not have the foul smelling mucous.

Postmortem Findings - In chicks there is yellowish cheesy plugs in the throat and swollen and pale kidneys. In larger birds there are swollen pale kidneys with maybe urate crystals in the tubes leaving the kidneys, fluid yolk or whole eggs in the abdominal cavity of hens.

Herbal Treatment

Put electrolytes in the drinking water and keep the birds warm and well fed, avoid crowding and watch for secondary bacterial infections particularly Air Sac disease. Survivors are permanently immune but become carriers and hens will normally return to production in 6 to 8 weeks but may never produce the same quality or quantity as before due to permanent ovary damage.

Give Echinacea for 2 weeks so as to build up the immune system and give plenty of garlic internally, fast for one day then give a laxative diet. Latter diet should include daily Cod Liver Oil (Vitamin A) and plenty of chopped onions and mustard greens. Give inhalations of

Eucalyptus oil turned into vapor in boiling water. I think Parsley would be a good herb to use here as its actions a expectorant, diuretic and antiseptic and it is also high in Vit C which would build up the immune system. One of the main reasons for this herb is because of its actions on the kidneys and especially the crystals found there. Other herbs to think of are Liquorice and Mullein. Also see Chickweed

Homoeopathic Treatment

Aconitum - Always give at the first signs of a respiratory problem and you may stop the disease from progressing. Eyes red and inflamed with swollen lids, watering. Running nose and sneezing, coughing. There may be fever and thirst and usually there is restlessness and anxiety.

Ant Tart - Moist cough with threatened pulmonary edema. Rattling sounds may be heard in the chest, respirations increased.

Arsenicum - Discharge is acrid, swollen eyelids with tears, chest wheezy and coughing, thirst for small quantities often, restless, irritable, worse after midnight, better for warmth.

Bryonia - Cough hard and dry, pleura becomes affected, relief from pressure over the ribs. Condition is worse from movement, animal rests on painful side.

Dulcamara - Condition has origins from damp surroundings and coughing worse after exertion. Loose rattling cough and nasal discharge. Can be given alternating with Sulphur 6C.

Kali Bich - Mucous of a tough stringy nature colored yellow, phlegm in bronchial tubes difficult to expel, discharges with edema of the eyelids, catarrhal inflammation of the sinuses, papular eruptions with ulcers, nasal discharge, weakness, Symptoms worse in the mornings, worse from cold, better for heat.

Air Sac Disease

This is a common disease which affects the respiratory system and has a incubation period of 6 to 21 days. The cause is from the bacteria Escherichia Coli and Mycoplasma Gallisepticum which is highly contagious and can have a mortality rate of up to 30%. This disease can happen often after vaccination.

Symptoms

In young birds 5 to 12 weeks old there can be coughing, rattling, nasal discharge, breathing difficulty, loss of appetite, rapid loss of weight, stunted growth and standing around with the eyes closed.

Resembles - Chronic Respiratory Disease except this affects older birds and the symptoms are usually milder.

Postmortem Findings - Thick mucous in nasal passages and throat. Cloudy air sacs containing cheesy material. Transparent film covering liver and heart.

Herbal Treatment

Give Echinacea for 2 weeks so as to build up the immune system and give plenty of garlic internally, fast for one day then give a laxative diet. Keep birds warm. Latter diet should include daily Cod Liver Oil (Vitamin A required by mucous membranes) and plenty of chopped onions and mustard greens (contain a lot of sulphur). Give inhalations of Eucalyptus oil turned into vapor in boiling water. As you can see again our main remedy is Garlic, the reason for this is that Garlic leaves the body via the mucous membranes, so as it is leaving its main actions as a herb are taking place with the one we are counting on being Antibiotic. Garlic is very high in sulphur so think of it working as a Sulphur antibiotic. Now imagine what we are doing. The air sacs in birds take up a very large area and are covered with mucous membranes from which our Garlic is now exiting. To prove to you how good this action is take a Garlic oil capsule and put it on the ground, next take off your sock and crush it with your heel and in a few moments you will be able to taste the Garlic exiting the mucous membranes in your mouth. Other herbs to look at are Plantain, Fenugreek, Liquorice and Mullein.

Homoeopathic Treatment

Use Potencies 6C to 30C

Aconitum - Always give at the first signs of a respiratory problem and you may stop the disease from progressing. Eyes red and inflamed with swollen lids, watering. Running nose and sneezing.

There may be fever and thirst and usually there is restlessness and anxiety.

Arsenicum - Discharge is acrid, swollen eyelids with tears, chest wheezy, thirst for small quantities, restless, irritable, worse after midnight. Dose every 2 hours for 4 doses.

Allium Cepa 6C - Discharge bland and watery, eyes red and watery and showing photophobia. Dose hourly for 4 doses.

Mercurius Sol - Much sneezing, nostrils raw with yellow greenish foul smelling discharge. Swollen eyelids with discharge.

Dulcamara - Sneezing is severe and eyes and nose are generally streaming, there can be a loose cough, the condition is usually caught from the wet and cold. Alternates well with Hepar Sulph.

Hepar Sulph 200C - Sneezing with ulceration of the nostrils, discharge thick and purulent, foul smelling, sensitive to pain, resents cold wind. Dose 3 times daily for 2 days. Is the best remedy where there has been partial relief from other remedies but not a full cure.

Kali Bich - Mucous of a tough stringy nature colored yellow, phlegm in bronchial tubes difficult to expel, discharges with edema of the eyelids, catarrhal inflammation of the sinuses, papular eruptions with ulcers, nasal discharge, weakness, Symptoms worse in the mornings, worse from cold, better for heat.

Wet Pox or Fowl Pox

This can also be known as Fowl Diphtheria and is different from the Dry Pox which attacks the outside skin and also less common then Dry Pox though sometimes both forms can turn up in the same animal. Here the upper respiratory tract is affected and there is a incubation period of 4 to 14 days. Progression of the disease and spread is slow and the disease lasts 3 to 5 weeks in individual birds and can have a mortality rate of up to 50%. The cause of the disease is a virus, the same one that causes Dry Pox and transmission is through skin wounds from fighting or mosquitoes.

Symptoms

In birds of all ages except newly hatched chicks there can be a transparent whitish wart like or scabby bumps on the face, comb and eyes (can cause blindness) and symptom similar to Dry Pox. In the

Diphtheritic form of the disease there are yellowish raised necrotic patches in the mouth and throat. They are firmly adherent to the mucous membrane and may become so extensive as to interfere with eating and breathing. Sometime these can be removed manually.

Resembles - Infectious Laryngotracheitis.

Postmortem Findings - Yellowish or brownish cheesy masses in mouth, upper throat and wind pipe anchored by cheese like roots.

Herbal Treatment

Give Echinacea for 2 weeks so as to build up the immune system along with Garlic applied internally and externally as a lotion on the affected areas. Fast for one day and then follow with a laxative diet. Juliette de Bairacli Levy says give 2 drops of Eucalyptus oil a day per hen. Other herbs to look at are chickweed to be used internally and externally and Thuja externally (for wart like growths) also think of Calendula externally. Look to the other disease write ups to find herbs covering the more respiratory type symptoms. After a cure all poultry must be moved and their home disinfected. Specific herbs for Diphtheria are Golden Seal and Lavender though I am not sure how they will handle these the death rate for this disease calls for their use. Chickweed externally may be useful. Shitake should be thought of as well because of its anti-viral and immune boosting properties.

Homoeopathic Treatment

Use Potencies 6C to 30C

Aconitum - Always give at the first signs of a respiratory problem and you may stop the disease from progressing. Eyes red and inflamed with swollen lids, watering. Running nose and sneezing. There may be fever and thirst and usually there is restlessness and anxiety.

Arsenicum - Discharge is acrid, swollen eyelids with tears, chest wheezy, thirst for small quantities often, restless, irritable, worse after midnight, skin may be dry and scaly with feather loss and pustules.

Mercurius Sol - Much sneezing, nostrils raw with yellow greenish foul smelling discharge. Swollen eyelids with discharge. There can be skin eruptions and itching, worse at night.

Rhus Tox - Restless, irritable, pox like eruptions, blistery eruptions, watery inflamed eyes, sneezing, nasal discharge, head and face have a swollen appearance, dry cough, very itchy.

Diptherinum 30C Nosode - Breath and discharge from throat, nose and mouth is offensive, bleeding from nose, extremities cold with marked debility, lies in semi stupid condition, eyes dull, pulse weak and rapid.

Chronic Respiratory Disease.

In turkeys this disease is called Infectious Sinusitis. Common worldwide but more so in winter and large commercial flocks and has a incubation period of 6 to 21 days. The disease spreads slowly and lasts longer in colder weather. The cause is Mycoplasma Gallissepticum Bacteria often aided by Escherichia Coli and or a Reovirus and is often seen in combination with Cholera, Infectious Bronchitis, Infectious Coryza, and can often follow after vaccinations. Mortality is usually low except in young birds.

Symptoms

In broilers 3 to 8 weeks old there is a drop in feed consumption and slow growth. In growing or mature birds there may be no symptoms or droopiness, coughing, sneezing, rattling, gurgling, swelling of the sinuses of the face, swollen face, nasal discharge, ruffled feathers, frothy and runny eyes, squeaky crow, drop in laying, loss of appetite, loss of weight, yellowish droppings.

Resembles - Most of the other respiratory diseases but spreads slower.

Postmortem Findings - Thick mucous in nasal passages and throat, cheesy material in air sacs, thickened heart sack and a transparent covering the liver.

Herbal Treatment

Give Echinacea for 2 weeks so as to build up the immune system and give plenty of garlic internally, fast for one day then give a laxative diet. Keep birds warm. Latter diet should include daily Cod Liver Oil (Vitamin A required by mucous membranes) and plenty of chopped onions and mustard greens (sulphur). Give inhalations of Eucalyptus oil turned into vapour in boiling water. As you can see again our main remedy is Garlic, the reason for this is that in CRD the whole of the respiratory system is involved, all of the lungs and all of the air sacs. This disease could be the cause of all the above diseases or it could be a opportunist who will come after the above diseases when the immunity is lowered. Other herbs to look at are Plantain, Fenugreek, Liquorice and Mullein. Vitamin C would also help to boost the immune system.

Homoeopathic Treatment

Aconitum - Always give at the first signs of a respiratory problem and you may stop the disease from progressing. Eyes red and inflamed with swollen lids, watering. Running nose and sneezing, coughing. There may be fever and thirst and usually there is restlessness and anxiety.

Ant Tart - Moist cough with threatened pulmonary oedema, Rattling sounds may be herd in the chest, respirations increased.

Arsenicum - Discharge is acrid, swollen eyelids with tears, chest wheezy and coughing, thirst for small quantities often, restless, irritable, worse after midnight, better for warmth.

Allium Cepa 6C - Discharge bland and watery, eyes red and watery and showing photophobia. Dose hourly for 4 doses.

Bryonia - Cough hard and dry, pleura becomes effected, relief from pressure over the ribs. Condition is worse from movement, animal rests on painful side.

Dulcamara - Condition has origins from damp surroundings, coughing worse after exertion. Loose rattling cough and nasal discharge. Can be given alternating with Sulphur 6C.

Kali Bich - Mucous of a tough stringy nature coloured yellow, phlegm in bronchial tubes difficult to expel, discharges with odema of the eyelids, catarrhal inflammation of the sinuses, papular eruptions with ulcers, nasal discharge, weakness. Symptoms worse in the mornings, worse from cold, better for heat.

Mercurius Sol - Much sneezing, nostrils raw with yellow greenish foul smelling discharge. Swollen eyelids with discharge.

The Digestive System

Crop Bound

Also called crop impaction and pendulous crop. Causes may be genetic, injury, fungal infection, or insufficient food. Other causes, may be from indigestion caused from Coccidiosis, worms, fibrous vegetable matter, pieces of wire or twine etc. Also blockages of the gizzard or intestines from tumors, worms, retained egg yolks etc.

Symptoms

In mature birds a distended sour smelling crop filled with feed and roughage. The crop feels hard when pressed with fingers and there may be emaciation. The hen shows a disinclination to eat and there is often a staggering gait.

Postmortem Findings - Sometimes sores in crop lining.

Resembles - Thrush except that in crop impaction birds appear healthy.

Herbal Treatment

Juliette de Bairacli Levy treats this condition with half a teaspoonful of Gentian Root powder brewed in a small cup of water then add a table spoon of milk and then 2 teaspoonfuls of olive oil. Divide into 2 parts and give the second part 2 hour after the first. A full teaspoon full of linseed oil is another remedy. Fasting and gentle manipulation generally cures.

A simple operation is the cutting open of the crop, removal of its contents, sprinkle the clean crop walls with one teaspoonful of black pepper, sew up with a ordinary needle and strong thread. Use a Calendula lotion on the wound to speed healing and sealing. Garlic internally could be used as a good antibiotic to protect the bird and wound.

Normal Treatment - Disinfect skin then slit through skin with sharp blade, pull skin aside and slit through crop, clean out crop, isolate bird and keep wound clean until it heals.

Homoeopathic Treatment

Nux Vom - Eating of indigestible foods, over eating, digestive disturbances and congestions. For sluggish Digestive systems combine with Carbo Veg.

Arsenicum Alb - There is great restlessness, great thirst for small quantities of water, loss of condition.

Coccidiosis

Common worldwide especially in warm humid weather. The cause can be from several different species of coccidial protozoan parasites that flourish in warm humid environments and survive for long periods outside the body, more than one species may infect a bird at any one time and the presence of coccidia does not always cause infection. Transmission is from droppings of effected birds. Affects the intestinal tract and has a incubation period of 5 days and then may progress to a chronic disease. 80 to 100 percent of the flock may be affected and the mortality rate may be high or low depending on the health before the onset.

Symptoms

In growing or semi mature birds there may be droopiness, faltering gait, huddling with ruffled feathers, loss of interest in water or feed, retarded growth or weight loss, there may be blood tinged or mucousy diarrhea, emaciation and dehydration, birds become depressed, wings droop and blood may appear in droppings. In mature birds there may be a drop in laying, thin breast, weak legs and sometimes diarrhea. In the yellow skinned breeds there is pale skin and comb.

Resembles - Infectious anemia, ulcerative enteritis, salmonellosis, worms and other enteric diseases.

Postmortem Findings - Varies depending on the species.

Herbal Treatment

Garlic is one of the main remedies especially because of its high sulphur and Vitamin C content. Given regularly it increases immunity and can be a preventative. Echinacea is another good one for not only does it boost the immune system but it is a antimicrobial as well.

Golden seal is useful against enteric protozoa eg coccidiosis and for improving digestive function in general but is not recommended for laying hens because of its action on the uterus but a few doses would not hurt. Barberry is another herb to think of because it shares some of the chemical ingredients of Golden Seal and has been used by itself to treat round worms. Black and Green tea are both strong tannins and have been shown to reduce worm burdens with the black tea better for small intestinal parasites including protozoa.

Juliette de Bairacli Levy treats this condition with a fast of a day on water only. She gives drops of senna brew with a tiny bit of ginger added usually a half desert spoon full dose, tea spoon full for chicks. One flaked clove of garlic is given per hen and the treatment is continued for about 10 days. In cases of severe exhaustion give drops of warm honey as this is a immediate restorative. Drops of sweet red wine are also lifesaving. Diet following the fast should be laxative. Bran and molasses mashes, plenty of green food especially chickweed, rue, mustard tops, comfrey, lettuce and all cresses. In Coccidiosis all poultry must be moved to entirely fresh land after cure and the old ground should be heavily limed. Fumigate the poultry places with burning cayenne pepper powder.

Pat Coleby says he had no more problems with Coccidiosis in his Goats after he planted some Mallow (Malva Plants) in the paddock which he says have a reputation of preventing this condition and also noticed that the stock which had the right amount of Copper supplemented seemed not to get the disease.

Homoeopathic Treatment

Aconitum - If seen in the early stages this remedy may help limit the disease process. Dose once every half hour for 4 doses.

Arsenicum Alb - This remedy should prove effective in the milder case showing diarrhoea and loss of condition. Dose 3 times daily for 4 days.

Ipecac - A good anti hemorrhagic remedy that appears to have a specific action on the intestine in the presence of protozoa. Dose 3 times daily for 5 days.

Mercurius Corr - This remedy is valuable where there is severe straining accompanied by dysenteric slimy stools. Dose 2 times daily for 5 days.

China 6C - This remedy will help restore strength after loss of body fluid following diarrhoea. Dose 3 times per day for 3 days.

Veratrum Alb - This remedy should help milder cases showing persistent diarrhea of a explosive type with threatened collapse. Dose 3 times daily for 5 days.

Simple Diarrhea

With the Homoeopathic Remedies use Aconite first so as to prevent it from becoming a more nasty disease especially if you think the condition was brought on by getting chilled. For more remedies look at the different conditions in this section and match the color of the stools.

Herbal Treatment

Treat the diarrhea with Slippery Elm, if there is lack of appetite mix the Slippery Elm with honey and water. Another herb that can be used for diarrhea brought on by chill is Ginger. The dried root is used to treat diarrhea associated with cold weather and cold damp conditions especially when you notice a drop in body temperature by finding cold feet and a cold comb.

Pasted Vent

This is also known as Vent Gleet. This condition is common in chicks but less so in mature birds. The cause is unknown but in chicks it may be from the rations or chilling and in Hens maybe a loss of muscle tone due to heredity weakness. Consider separating the sick individuals.

Symptoms

In chicks up to 10 days old droopiness, droppings sticking to vent. In laying hens there is a offensive odor and droppings stick to vent and feathers. In all there may be a yellow discharge from the vent fetid and gluey matting the feathers. Carefully pick away adhering matter and cull chicks that don't recover. Death is possible if vent gets sealed shut.

For prevention keep chicks warm and do not hatch eggs from effected Hens.

Resembles - In chicks Arizonosis and Paratyphoid.

Postmortem Findings - Distended rectum filled with droppings.

Herbal Treatment

Use Garlic as the main remedy and fast for a day and then give a laxative diet. Externally the vent should be cleaned with a lotion of Garlic and Calendula both powerful herbal disinfectants.

Chamomile Tea is useful for diarrhea in young birds where there have been disturbances, changes of routine and anxiety.

Homoeopathic Treatment

Aconite 30C- Diarrhea in the primary stage, at the beginning of acute cases that come on suddenly and violently, when it arises from taking cold, considerable fever, inflammation of the bowels, can be alternated with Nux Vom.

Nux Vom 12X - Discharges slimy and offensive with rumbling noises in the bowels and passing of wind, when there are symptoms of indigestion and when purging is alternated with constipation.

Arsenicum - For watery, slimy, greenish or brownish diarrhea, with or without gripping pains and can smell offensive, great rumbling in the bowels and flatulence, total loss of appetite and a marked prostration of strength, skin and extremities cold, great restlessness.

China 30C - Useful in chronic cases or when caused by hot weather and not of a inflammatory character, painless discharge, loss of appetite and strength. Yellow, brown watery stools. Can be used as a tonic when acute symptoms have passed away, evacuations consist partly of undigested food can be pain during discharge.

Bryonia - If the disorder has been brought on by a change of temperature especially from hot to cold, by drinking cold water or impure water, fasces are very watery and involuntary passed and may contain undigested food, can be alternating diarrhea and constipation.

Mercurius Cor - Frequent discharge of mucous tinged with blood or thin bloody and fetid stools, frequent urging to stool, redness and swollen appearance of the anus, symptoms worse at night.

Gelsemium - General state of exhaustion, copious yellow flow from relaxed uncontrolled anus. No appetite or thirst.

Campylobacteriosis (Hepatitis)

Also known as Avain Vibrionic Hepatitis. This condition is common worldwide especially on floor reared flocks. The disease has a 24 hour incubation period and mainly effects the intestines and liver. The cause is Campylobacter Fetus Jejuni bacteria that among birds only affects chickens. This bacteria survives well and can resist disinfectants and often occurs in combination with other diseases such as Mareks or Pox. Transmission is from droppings of infected carrier birds. The mortality rate of this disease is 10 to 15%.

Symptoms

In chicks up to 4 weeks old there can be depression, watery diarrhea, slow growth in the chronic condition and maybe death in the acute condition. In growing and mature birds there may be sudden death of apparently healthy birds or for the chronic symptoms there may be listlessness, scaly shrunken comb, weight loss and sometimes bloody diarrhea. In hens the only sign may be a 35% drop in egg production. Severely affected birds lose weight and are listless and roost or stand apart from the others. Their combs usually become dry, shrivelled and scaly. Bird less severely affected may appear normal.

Postmortem Findings - Intestines filled with mucous and watery fluid, pale watery bone marrow. Sometime green or brown stained liver with characteristic yellow star shaped patches.

Resembles - Black Head, Blue Comb, Infectious Anemia, Cholera, Typhoid, Ulcerative Enteritis.

Herbal Treatment

With liver problems the best way to start would be a fast so as to rest the liver and give it a chance to sort itself out. As this is a bacterial infection give Echinacea for 2 weeks and also Garlic to start on the battle with the causative bacterial agents. Dandelion and Milk Thistle are two good herbs to look at for serious liver problems. Astragalus can be given after Echinacea's time is up. Treat the diarrhea especially if it is blood with Slippery Elm, if there is lack of appetite mix the Slippery Elm with honey and water.

Homoeopathic Treatment

This will depend on the overall symptom picture but there are certain remedies that have a action on the liver and they include the following.

Aconite 30C - Give at the onset of the problem especially if it arises from cold or there is fever.

Chelidonium 6C - General lethargy yellowish tongue and discoloration of visible mucous membranes, eyes may be weepy, signs of stiffness or pain may be evident over the right shoulder region , stools are clay colored, touch and movement aggravate. Strong yellow discoloration of visible mucous membranes.

Aesculus 30C - Jaundice, the portal circulation becomes congested leading to signs of abdominal discomfort soon after eating, tenderness over the liver, stools are large and hard and the urine becomes discolored, there may be accompanying respiratory symptoms such as coughing up mucous.

Chamomilla 30C - Useful if there is general yellowness of the skin, restless, lying down and quickly getting up.

Lycopodium - A prominent liver remedy, inability to eat much at any one time, very little food appears to satisfy, all symptoms aggravated in the late afternoon and early evening, a good remedy for the old and for lean animals, stools are generally hard.

Mag Mur 30C - Enlargement of liver, jaundice and abdominal pain pronounced. Dose night and morning for 4 days.

China 30C - Weakness and debility, abdominal pain, stools yellow and fluid, increasing weakness. Dose every 3 hours for 4 doses.

Berberis Vulgaris 30C - Sluggish liver conditions with tenderness over lumber region. Skin yellowish, diarrhea symptoms present. Dose 3 times daily for 3 days.

Infectious Stunting Syndrome

Can also be known as Malabsorption Syndrome and Pale Bird Syndrome. This is a fairly new condition that appeared several years ago and affects the digestive system and seems to have a incubation period of 1 to 13 days and turns into a type of chronic disease. The cause is unknown though a virus is suspected and in reality it is probably a mixture of pathogens. The transmission is not known either but the incidence seems to be less in hygienically kept homes.

Symptoms

This disease is characterized by severe stunting of chicks arising very soon after they go in the broiler house. It is usually first noticeable at 10 days of age. Sometimes the condition is called Helicopter Disease because feathering is very bad and some of the wing feathers protrude Horizontality from the bird. By the killing age of 50 days the affected birds weight will be about half of the normal weight. Deaths are relatively few.

In 1 to 6 week old birds there can be uneven or seriously stunted growth, chick only reach half their normal size by 4 weeks of age. There may be pale skin, slow feather development, sometimes a protruding abdomen, undigested feed in the droppings, diarrhea, increased thirst, lameness or reluctance to walk. There is a 5 to 30 percent infection rate.

Postmortem Findings - Enlarged sometimes bloody stomach (proventriculus), pale distended intestines, small intestine filled with poorly digested feed, Sometimes the pancreas is thin, white and fibrous or can be grossly atrophied.

Resembles – Infectious Anemia and Runting Syndrome.

Herbal Treatment

The first herb to think of is Astragalus which should be given to all to build up their immune systems and to protect them from viruses, for the ones that are already sick they will have the extra benefits of a herb that gives them strength when they are run down and debilitated. This herb is also a digestive tonic and is used for wasting diseases. Meaning as though the Pancreas seems to be taking damage as confirmed in the postmortem and the undigested food in the stools we should look at the herb Golden Seal which has a strong action on this organ and is also a digestive tonic.

Other herbs to look at are Gentian as a digestive tonic and Chamomile whose antiinflammatory, antiseptic and antispasmodic action should help the intestine. Chamomile is a specific remedy for the Young.

Homoeopathic Treatment

Aconite 30C- Diarrhea in the primary stage, at the beginning of acute cases that come on suddenly and violently, when it arises from taking cold, considerable fever, inflammation of the bowels, can be alternated with Nux Vom. Dose - every half hour for 4 doses.

Nux Vom 12X - Discharges slimy and offensive with rumbling noises in the bowels and passing of wind, when there are symptoms of indigestion. Dose once every 2 hours.

Arsenicum - For watery, slimy, greenish or brownish diarrhea, with or without gripping pains and can smell offensive, great rumbling in the bowels and flatulence, total loss of appetite and a marked prostration of strength, skin and extremities cold, great restlessness.

China 30C - Useful in chronic cases or when caused by hot weather and not of a inflammatory character, painless discharge, loss of appetite and strength. Can be used as a tonic when acute symptoms have passed away, evacuations consist partly of undigested food , can be pain during discharge.

Bryonia 30C- If the disorder has been brought on by a change of temperature especially from hot to cold, by drinking cold water or impure water, fasces are very watery and involuntary passed and may contain undigested food, can be alternating diarrhea and constipation. Dose four times a day.

Chamomilla 30C- If there is pain just before a evacuation which is of a greenish color with phlegm.

Cholera

Can also be known as Avian Hemorrhagic Septicemia. This condition is more likely to happen in warm climates and free ranged birds and is more prevalent in the late summer, fall and winter.

The incubation period is 4 to 9 days and it is a acute disease that spreads rapidly and kills quickly.

The cause is the bacteria Pasteurella Multocida that affects a variety of birds. The bacteria can survive for one month in manure and 3 months in moist soil but can be destroyed by 10 minutes in sunlight and also easily destroyed by disinfectants. Transmission is from contact with mucous from the nose mouth or eyes which contaminates the water or by pecking at a carcass. There is no vaccination or treatment for this disease.

Symptoms

In mature birds or those approaching maturity there can be sudden death with hens found dead in the nesting boxes or symptoms of fever, loss of appetite, increased thirst, depression, drowsiness, ruffled feathers, head pale and drawn back, increased respiratory rate, mucous discharge from mouth and nose, watery white diarrhea latter becoming thick and greenish yellow, bluish comb and wattles and death can be within hours of the first symptoms. Survivors may recover and either eventually die from emaciation and dehydration or develop chronic cholera. Chronic Cholera may show as lesions such as localized swelling in joints, eyes, throat and wattles. Mortality can be 10 to 20% among mature birds to 45% overall. Below is another description of the disease which I have taken out of a well over a 100 year old Chicken Book. Symptoms - sad looks, lost appetite, weakness, staggering, thirst, hanging heads, in more advanced cases a tough mucous trickled from the bills which hang so low as to touch the ground, the comb becomes shrunken and of a bluish color while the diarrhea is violent and almost liquid looking yellowish or greenish and frothy and as the end approaches the eyes close.

Postmortem Findings - Nothing in cases of sudden death, otherwise blood in lungs and in fatty tissue of the abdomen, heart surrounded by a fluid containing cheesy flakes, swollen grayish liver (looks cooked) with smallish gray white spots. Sticky mucous in the digestive tract especially in the crop and intestines.

Resembles - Typhoid and poisoning.

Herbal Treatment

Give Astragalus, Echinacea and Garlic to all immediately. Use Homoeopathic Remedies on the infected chickens as they are faster acting. Use Aconite 30C Immediately.

Homoeopathic Treatment

Arsenicum - For watery, slimy, greenish or brownish diarrhea, with or without gripping pains and can smell offensive, great rumbling in the bowels and flatulence, total loss of appetite and a marked prostration of strength, fever, skin and extremities cold , great restlessness, great thirst for small quantities of water. Dose - every hour for 4 doses.

Arsenicum Iod - Similar to the above but with more Respiratory Problems.

Aconite - Dairrhoea in the primary stage, at the beginning of acute cases that come on suddenly and violently, restlessness and anxiety, when it arises from taking cold, considerable fever, inflammation of the bowels.

Veratrum Alb - Specific for Cholera often after Arsenicum, septic feverish states, extreme coldness, blueness, weakness, very similar in symptoms to Arsenicum.

Cuprum - Is another specific for Cholera with similar symptoms to the above but is more of a violent spasmodic and cramping and convulsing type of remedy, pale bluish, craves cool drink, colic with diarrhea.

Paratyphoid

Common worldwide and affects the digestive system or entire body. Has a incubation period of 5 days. The cause is from a Salmonella bacteria that resides in soil and litter. In some places this is a reportable disease. See **Note** at bottom of write up.

Symptoms

In chicks up to 5 weeks there could be death at the time of hatching or depression, weakness, poor growth, drooping wings, decreased appetite, increased thirst, chirping or peeping sounds, huddled around heat with feathers ruffled, eyes closed, head down, sometimes swollen joints, swelling or blindness in one or both eyes, watery diarrhea with pasting and dehydration.

In adults carriers there may be no symptoms or reduced egg production, purplish head, comb and wattles.

Postmortem Findings - Usually inconclusive though there may be a swollen liver.

Resembles - Typhoid, Pullorum and Infectious Synovitis when the joints are swollen.

Herbal Treatment

Think of Echinacea and Garlic straight away as this is a bacterial infection also think of Burdock as a blood cleanser. After Echinacea's 2 weeks are up think of Astragalus. The following comes out of Juliette de Bairacli Levy book and is her treatment for Typhoid in poultry. She believes the condition is caused by too much artificial feeding and a dirty blood stream. Her treatment is fasting with Garlic. Also half a teaspoon of lemon juice per hen twice daily, dilute with the same quantity with a brew of Sage (Nervine, Blood Cleanser). Add finely cut Rue and Sage leaves to bran and molasses mash. Transfer all poultry to new ground.

Homoeopathic Treatment

Aconite - Diarrhea in the primary stage, at the beginning of acute cases that come on suddenly and violently, restlessness and anxiety, when it arises from taking cold, considerable fever, inflammation of the bowels.

Arsenicum - For watery, slimy, greenish or brownish diarrhea, with or without gripping pains and can smell offensive, great rumbling in the bowels and flatulence, total loss of appetite and a marked prostration of strength, fever, skin and extremities cold , great restlessness, great thirst for small quantities of water. Dose every hour for 4 doses.

Baptisia - Low potencies of this remedy can raise the immunities of those not infected and give the infected ones a high potency. This remedy is the specific for Typhoid. Low fevers, septic conditions of the blood, extreme prostration, all secretions are offensive, mental confusion , perfect indifference or stupor, no appetite constant desire for water, stools offensive, thin dark and bloody, pain over liver region, difficult breathing, burning and heat in the skin.

Phosphoric Acid - Mental debility followed by physical debility, hemorrhages in Typhoid, apathetic, indifferent, distended abdomen, diarrhea white watery and involuntary, weak extremities, pain in joints, low types of fever, better from warmth and worse from exertion.

Rhus Tox - Typhoid type fever with marked joint pains, hot painful swelling of joints, septicemia, extreme restlessness with much changing of position, eyes can be swollen and red, swollen face and glands, great thirst, colic, frothy, slimy foul smelling stools, better warmth.

Note

There are 2 forms of Salmonella species that are specific to Poultry they are Salmonella Pullorum also known as Bacillary White Diarrhea (the next write up) and Salmonella Gallinarum which is known as Fowl typhoid. There are many other forms of Salmonella way over 2000 have been found and they all may potentially effect poultry and those that do are generally termed Avain Paratyphoid.

Pullorum

Also known as bacillary White Diarrheal. Affects mostly chickens and Turkeys though any fowl may get infected. The cause is from the bacteria Salmonella Pullorum which can survive for years in dry litter but is easily destroyed by cleaning and disinfectants. Transmission is primarily from the egg though can also be from infected breeders to chicks or spread from chick to chick. In some places this is a reportable disease and the survivors are culled. Humans eating the contaminated meat can get a acute intestinal infection with high fever and prostration. Do not keep recovered Hens for egg production.

Symptoms

This disease is highly fatal to young chicks and poults but mature birds are more resistant. In chicks up to 4 weeks old there can be sudden death or loss of appetite, sleepiness, weakness, huddling near heat, swollen hock joints, white or greenish brown pasty diarrheal, sometimes gasping, shrill peeping or chirping while trying to expel droppings, labored breathing, ruffled feathers, uneven growth among survivors.

In mature birds there may be no signs or loss of appetite, increased thirst, sometime pale shriveled comb, green diarrhea and a drop in egg production.

Mortality can be up to 90% in chicks increasing on the fourth or fifth day and peaking at 2 to 3 weeks of age.

Postmortem Findings - In chicks there may be cheesy material in abdominal cavity or ceca, enlarged liver, kidneys, heart and spleen, small white or grey nodules up to pea size in liver, heart, gizzard, intestine and lungs.

In adult birds there may be enlarged liver, heart, spleen and kidneys, swollen ceca or oviduct filled with firm cheesy material.

In Hens there may be brownish or greenish shriveled yolks, yolk material in abdominal cavity.

In Cocks there may be shriveled testicles.

Resembles - Paratyphiod and white diarrhea due to simple chilling.

Herbal Treatment

Treat as for Coccidiosis but give 3 times daily a small feed of powdered slippery Elm bark with honey and warm milk. Concentrate mainly on Echinacea, Garlic and have a good look at the herbs Golden Seal and maybe latter Gentian. Much attention should be paid to disinfection of the houses and runs.

Homoeopathic Treatment

Aconite - Diarrhea in the primary stage, at the beginning of acute cases that come on suddenly and violently, restlessness and anxiety, when it arises from taking cold, considerable fever, inflammation of the bowels.

Arsenicum - For watery, slimy, greenish or brownish diarrhea, with or without gripping pains and can smell offensive, great rumbling in the bowels and flatulence, total loss of appetite and a marked prostration of strength, fever, skin and extremities cold , great restlessness, great thirst for small quantities of water. Dose every hour for 4 doses.

Baptisia - Low potencies of this remedy can raise the immunities of those not infected and give the infected ones a high potency. This remedy is the specific for Typhoid. Low fevers, septic conditions of the blood, extreme prostration, all secretions are offensive, mental confusion , perfect indifference or stupor, no appetite constant desire for water, stools offensive, thin dark and bloody, pain over liver region, difficult breathing, burning and heat in the skin.

Phosphoric Acid - Mental debility followed by physical debility, hemorrhages in Typhoid, apathetic, indifferent, distended abdomen, diarrhea white watery and involuntary, weak extremities, pain in joints, low types of fever, better from warmth and worse from exertion.

Rhus Tox - Typhoid type fever with marked joint pains, hot painful swelling of joints, septicemia, extreme restlessness with much changing of position, eyes can be swollen and red, swollen face and glands, great thirst, colic, frothy, slimy foul smelling stools, better warmth.

The Nervous System

Botulism

Also called food poisoning and limbernec. The cause is the bacteria Clostridium Botulinum which is a soil borne bacteria that produces toxins when they multiply in decaying vegetable or animal matter. The transmission is from consuming decaying organic matter or those who have such as maggots or beetles or feeding on rotten animal tissue or drinking contaminated water. The intensity of the disease is dose related. Free range are affected more, keep them away from the compost heap.

Symptoms

Symptoms are dose related. In birds of all ages there can be sudden death or leg weakness and drowsiness followed by a progressive flaccid (not rigid) paralysis of the legs, wings and neck with difficulty in swallowing. The feathers may be loose and ruffled and there may be raised hackles on cocks. There may be lying on the side without stretched neck and eyes partly closed. Sometimes there is trembling, diarrhea, coma and death due to heart and or respiratory failure.

Postmortem Findings - None obvious

Resembles - Tick paralysis while mild Botulism resembles Marek's Disease.

Herbal Treatment

Use Garlic as a anti-bacterial and Rosemary for its antibacterial and paralysis actions. Grapefruit seed extract is the only known herb to affect this strain of bacteria.

Homoeopathic Treatment

Gelsemium - Has a affinity for the nervous system where it produces various degrees of motor paralysis, loss of power occurs in muscles causing trembling and weakness of limbs, incoordination of movement then, general prostration, there may be difficulty in swallowing.

Lathyrus Sativa - Effects the bottom column of the spinal cord producing paralysis in the lower extremities, rigidity of muscles develop producing a weak tottery gait, there may be distress in breathing if these nerves become involved, difficulty in swallowing, much weakness and heaviness.

Curare 30C – (Arrow Poison). For milder cases showing muscular stiffness with difficulty in walking preceded by trembling of limbs, may be difficulty in breathing, worse from dampness and cold weather.

Coniun Mac 200C - A suitable remedy when paralytic symptoms are seen mainly in the lower limbs. The bird is sometimes unable to rise, the paralysis is ascending, eyes may be watery, difficult gait, trembling, loss of strength, good for treating tumors.

Plumbum Met 30C - This is also a good remedy for general paralysis of limb muscles especially the fore limbs, paralysis can be preceded by loss of sensation in the affected part, nerve pains, there can be convulsions, rapid emaciation, depression, good for treating tumors.

Marek's Disease

This disease is common worldwide but less so in bantams. The disease has a incubation period of 2 weeks and is caused by a Herpes virus that may result in death or severe production loss. The disease is highly contagious and can be spread by carrier birds and infected birds by the dust of their dander and feathers being inhaled as the virus is concentrated in the feather follicles. The virus can survive for years in dust and litter. Turkeys carry a related though harmless virus that keeps Marek,s virus from causing tumors.

Symptoms

The disease can be seen in two forms one that attacks the nerves while the other form produces tumors. Young birds are the most susceptible to infection and most deaths occur between 10 and 24 weeks of age.

In the tumor type of disease lesions are most commonly associated with the gonads, liver, spleen and kidneys however other such organs such as the lungs, heart and musculature are commonly involved. The disease is often acute with apparently healthy birds dyeing very rapidly with massive internal tumors. This form may produce severe losses in pullets. As this disease is seen often with Coccidiosis there may be some relationship between the two.

The nerve type form is the classical type with the paralysis.

In chicks over 3 weeks old they grow thin while eating well, deaths start at 8 to 10 weeks and persist until 20 to 25 weeks.

In maturing birds 6 to 9 months old there may be enlarged reddened feather follicles or white bumps on the skin that scab over with a brown crust, stilted gate or lack of co-ordination, pale skin, wing or leg paralysis, when both legs are paralysed one points back and the other points forward and this is the classic sign of the disease, sometimes there is rapid weight loss, gapping or gasping, transient paralysis lasting 1 or 2 days, dehydration, death due to inability to get to food and water or trampling.

The percentage affected can be 30 to 50 percent in unvaccinated flocks and less than 5% in vaccinated flocks while mortality in the infected can be nearly 100%.

Postmortem Findings - In cases of sudden death there have been found massive tumors especially along the spinal column, otherwise enlarged nerves with nodules usually on one side. Tumors in testes or ovary take on a cauliflower look, solidified lungs, extremely enlarged liver, spleen or kidneys with greyish white soft areas.

Resembles - Lymphoid leukosis and Botulism.

Herbal Treatment

As this is a fast acting disease herbs may not have enough time to do their work but the ones to consider are Echinacea so as to prime the immune system and as this is a virus we will concentrate on antivirals such as Garlic and two other herbs which are specific to the Herpes Virus St John's Wort and Lemon Balm. I don't know if these have been used in poultry before but in a disease as nasty as this I think it is well worth the risk. You could always experiment on half the causalities.

With the Lemon Balm if you can't get it in herb form you could get the essential oil and dilute it and rub it into the feet and comb and it will get into the blood stream this way. Another important herb to add to the above is Rosemary as it is a Nervine, antispasmodic painkiller used for paralysis.

Burdock might be worth trying as it is anti-tumor and a blood cleanser.

For this condition Juliette de Bairacli Levy says give a fasting and laxative diet as stated for Coccidiosis. Give plenty of molasses in the diet and also kelp powder and aromatic herbs such as Thyme, Rosemary and Dill. Give Garlic.

Homoeopathic Treatment

In cases not too far advanced the following remedies will be of value.

Gelsemium - Has an affinity for the nervous system where it produces various degrees of motor paralysis, loss of power occurs in muscles causing trembling and weakness of limbs, incoordination of movement then, general prostration, there may be difficulty in swallowing.

Lathyrus Sativa - Effects the bottom column of the spinal cord producing paralysis in the lower extremities, rigidity of muscles develop producing a weak tottery gait, there may be distress in breathing if these nerves become involved, difficulty in swallowing, much weakness and heaviness.

Curare 30C - Arrow Poison. For milder cases showing muscular stiffness with difficulty in walking preceded by trembling of limbs, may be difficulty in breathing, worse from dampness and cold weather.

Coniun Mac 200C - A suitable remedy when paralytic symptoms are seen mainly in the lower limbs. The bird is sometimes unable to rise, the paralysis is ascending, eyes may be watery, difficult gait, trembling, loss of strength, good for treating tumors.

Plumbum Met 30C - This is also a good remedy for general paralysis of limb muscles especially the fore limbs, paralysis can be preceded by loss of sensation in the affected part, nerve pains, there can be convulsions, rapid emaciation, depression, good for treating tumors.

Newcastle Disease

This is a reportable disease that affects chickens and turkeys. Also known as poultry plague. Rare but worldwide especially in young concentrated and confined flocks. The incubation period is 2 to 15 days and it spreads rapidly running through the flock in 3 to 4 days and lasts for 3 to 4 weeks. The cause is from a Paramyxovirus that can survive for 30 days outside the system but is very sensitive to sunlight.

Symptoms

Affects the respiratory and nervous system and sometimes also the digestive system. The disease often first shows as a common cold then a unusual dripping discharge from the beak begins followed by a rapid death. In all ages there is a sudden high rate of death without symptoms. In chicks there may gasping, sneezing, coughing, slow growth, drooping wings, dragging legs, sometimes twisted head and neck, circling, somersaulting, walking backwards and paralysis.

In mature birds there may be listlessness, rapid or difficult breathing, progressive weakness, near total cessation of laying within 3 days followed by loss of coordination, loss of appetite, muscular tremors, twisted neck, wing and leg paralysis, sometimes watery greenish blood stained diarrhea, swollen blackish eyes with a straw colored fluid draining from the eyes and nose, death within 2 to 3 days. Mortality is usually 50% in adults and 90% in young birds.

Postmortem - Yellow patches on the roof of the mouth, large and small reddish brown spots or blotches (hemorrhages) in the upper and lower digestive tract, over abdominal fat and on the ovary.

Resembles - Blackhead, Cholera, Coccidiosis, Thrush and Infectious Laryngotracheitis.

Herbal Treatment

I would approach this condition the same as Mareks Disease. For this condition Juliette de Bairacli Levy says give a fasting and laxative diet as stated for Coccidiosis. Wash out the beaks with diluted eucalyptus lotion. A well proved Turkish peasant treatment is ground raw garlic mixed with vinegar, 2 teaspoonful of herb to 1 of vinegar twice daily poured down the beak in half teaspoonful doses. Also olive oil is given night and morning. Honey can also be given.

Homoeopathic Treatment

Aconite - At the beginning of acute cases that come on suddenly and violently thee will be restlessness and anxiety, when it arises from taking cold, considerable fever, coryza with sneezing.

Arsenicum - For watery, slimy, greenish or brownish diarrhea, with or without gripping pains and can smell offensive, great rumbling in the bowels and flatulence, total loss of appetite and a marked prostration of strength, fever, skin and extremities cold , great restlessness, great thirst for small quantities of water. Dose - every hour for 4 doses.

Baptisia - Low fevers, septic conditions of the blood, extreme prostration, all secretions are offensive, mental confusion , perfect indifference or stupor, no appetite constant desire for water, stools offensive, thin dark and bloody, pain over liver region, difficult breathing, burning and heat in the skin.

Gelsemium - Has a affinity for the nervous system where it produces various degrees of motor paralysis, loss of power occurs in muscles causing trembling and weakness of limbs, incoordination of movement, general prostration, there may be difficulty in swallowing.

Lathyrus Sativa - Effects the bottom column of the spinal cord producing paralysis in the lower extremities, rigidity of muscles develop producing a weak tottery gait, there may be distress in breathing if these nerves become involved, difficulty in swallowing, much weakness and heaviness,

Curare 30C – (Arrow Poison). For milder cases showing muscular stiffness with difficulty in walking preceded by trembling of limbs, may be difficulty in breathing,, worse from dampness and cold weather.

The Muscular Skeletal System

Staphylococcic Arthritis

Common worldwide and affects the joints and the entire body when it is septicemic.

This condition affects chickens but there is a greater incidence of it in Turkeys. The septicemic form has a incubation period of 2 to 3 days. The cause is the bacteria Staphylococcus Alureus which is common in the poultry environment. Transmission is through bacteria entering the body through wounds.

Symptoms

This can be a acute (septicemic form) or chronic (arthritis) disease. In all ages there may be a fever, reluctance to move, ruffled feathers, depression, swollen joints that are hot to touch, resting on hocks and keel, chronic lameness and death. The main signs to look for are depression, diarrhea and swollen joints. More chronic cases show lameness and loss of condition. Death due to cannibalism occurs commonly in affected turkeys.

Postmortem Findings - Joints especially the hock and surrounding area are inflamed and contain whitish fleck filled pus that appears cheesy in a advanced condition. Sometimes there is a swollen and spotted spleen.

Resembles - Synovitis, viral arthritis except here the fluid surrounding the joints is yellowish or pinkish.

Herbal Treatment

Start the treatment with Echinacea and Garlic and after 2 weeks replace the Echinacea with Astragalus. Other herbs to look at are Celery Seed so as to remove the acids and wastes, this herb works well with Dandelion Root which balances its diuretic action and has its own specific action on arthritis. The last herb to look at is Burdock which is a Anti-bacterial blood cleanser along with being a good herb for arthritis which should work well with the Garlic in fighting the Septicemia part of this disease.

Homoeopathic Treatment

Aconite - At the beginning of acute cases that come on suddenly and violently, restlessness and anxiety, when it arises from taking cold, joints become swollen and hot.

Colchicum - Where the joint swelling is red or pale with extreme tenderness to touch, a tendency to shift about from joint to joint, pains worse motion, gout, great prostration of the muscular system, dysentery, more indicated in the smaller joints.

Rhus Tox 6C - Indicated when the animal gains relief from movement even though the initial movement is painful, symptoms may be more on the left side of the body then the right, indicated when severe wetting or prolong dampness is associated with the onset of the symptoms. Dose is twice daily for 21 days.

Bryonia 6C - Movement is resented when Bryonia is indicated. The animal will seek to lie on the affected muscles and pressure on them gives ease, warmth is usually useful also. Good for septicaemia. Dose twice daily for 15 days.

Causticum 12C - This remedy is associated with a accompanying contraction of tendons and a stiffness of muscles, warmth gives relief, more adaptable to the older patient with unsteadiness of gait. Dose is twice a day for 14 days.

Formic Acid 6X - Stiffness in joints, right side mostly affected, pains worse motion, better pressure, weakness of lower extremities, stiff and contracted joints.

Viral Arthritis

Fairly rare and the affected parts are the joints and tendons. The disease has a incubation period of 1 to 13 days and can be either acute or chronic. The cause of this disease is a Avian Reovirus that only effects chickens and is transmitted by contact with infected birds and is highly infectious. Recovered birds can be disease carriers for the next 2 months. Mildly infected birds recover in 4 to 6 weeks. The mortality rate can be 2 to 10% in young birds.

Symptoms

In young birds mainly of the heavy breeds 4 to 16 weeks old there may be lameness. In mature birds there may be bowed or straddled legs which can go undetected. In severe outbreaks there may be lameness, reduced weight gains and a increased number of stunted birds. Lesions of the disease are generally seen in the hock joints and tendons associated with them.

Postmortem Findings - Hocks and associated tendons are sometimes surrounded by a yellow or pinkish sticky fluid. Whitish foci of necrosis are sometimes seen in the heart muscle.

Resembles - Staphylococcic Arthritis or a simple leg injury.

Herbal Treatment

Start the treatment with Echinacea and Garlic and as this is a Viral infection think of Shitake Mushrooms. After 2 weeks replace the Echinacea with Astragalus. Other herbs to look at are Burdock and maybe Dandelion Root.

Homoeopathic Treatment

Aconite - At the beginning of acute cases that come on suddenly and violently, restlessness and anxiety, when it arises from taking cold, joints become swollen and hot.

Colchicum - Where the joint swelling is red or pale with extreme tenderness to touch, a tendency to shift about from joint to joint, pains worse motion, gout, great prostration of the muscular system, dysentery, more indicated in the smaller joints.

Rhus Tox 6C - Indicated when the animal gains relief from movement even though the initial movement is painful, symptoms may be more on the left side of the body then the right, indicated when severe wetting or prolonged dampness is associated with the onset of the symptoms. Dose is twice daily for 21 days.

Bryonia 6C - Movement is resented when Bryonia is indicated. The animal will seek to lie on the affected muscles and pressure on them gives ease, warmth is usually useful also. Good for septicemia. Dose twice daily for15 days.

Causticum 12C - This remedy is associated with a accompanying contraction of tendons and a stiffness of muscles, warmth gives relief, more adaptable to the older patient with unsteadiness of gait. Dose is twice a day for 14 days.

Formic Acid 6X - Stiffness in joints, right side mostly affected, pains worse motion, better pressure, weakness of lower extremities, stiff and contracted joints.

Gout

This can be sporadic and may be caused by nutrition from feeding to much protein or could be caused by kidney problems.

Symptoms

There may be enlarged foot joints with pasty white urate deposits easily seen through the skin.

Postmortem Findings - White tissue surrounding joints with white semi fluid deposits.

Resembles - No other disease.

Herbal Treatment

Insure that there is plenty of water so the urates can be flushed through the system and that the water is fresh and clean. If they are on bore water change it to fresh as our top priority now is to take as much work of the kidney as we can. Next is to change the diet by decreasing the protein concentration. The herb Gentian could be used as a digestive tonic as it helps to break down proteins along with Burdock which helps with digestion and kidney function along with all its other jobs. Dandelion Root and Celery Seed should also be thought of along with Couch Grass which cleans out gravel and stones in the kidneys and urinary system.

Homoeopathic Treatment

Colchicum - Where the joint swelling is red or pale with extreme tenderness to touch, a tendency to shift about from joint to joint, pains worse motion, gout, great prostration of the muscular system, dysentery, more indicated in the smaller joints.

Rhus Tox 6C - Indicated when the animal gains relief from movement even though the initial movement is painful, symptoms may be more on the left side of the body then the right, indicated when severe wetting or prolonged dampness is associated with the onset of the symptoms. Dose is twice daily for 21 days.

Bryonia 6C - Movement is resented when Bryonia is indicated. The animal will seek to lie on the affected muscles and pressure on them gives ease, warmth is usually useful also. Good for septicaemia. Dose twice daily for15 days.

Nat Phos and Nat Sulph 6X - These are Biochemic Cell Salts which remove acid and metabolic wastes from the body. Known as Cell Salts and are found in most Chemists and Health Shops.

Broken Leg

This can be common in poultry especially when they are confined. Make some wooden splints and bandage them firmly to the leg once you have set the leg. Another good alternative is to use a plastic syringe, pull and throw away the plunger then cut off the top and bottom then cut down the side. Line with cotton wool and use as a splint. Use a elastic type of bandage and put the bird somewhere that you can observe because with fractures the leg can swell and it the bandages are tight circulation will be cut off. Get some Comfrey leaves and dice them up finely and make a cold brew of them and put the bird's leg in it 3 times a day. If there are lacerations with the fracture you could make a lotion from Comfrey and Calendula together and soak the splint with this. Be careful if you use wood that it doesn't swell and tighten the bandage. Also give 1 teaspoonful of Comfrey Brew night and morning. Leave the splint on for 15 to 20 days or longer if it is a clumsy bird. Larger birds like the Turkey leave on for a month.

Homoeopathic Treatment

Arnica 6C- For the shock and bruised sore pains. Arnica cream can also be applied as long as the skin is not broken.

Calc Phos 6X - Helps in nutrition especially of the bones and promotes the knitting together of the bones. Helps fractures heal much faster. Can be used in alternation with Symphytum.

Ledum 6C - Take after arnica 4 hourly or 3 times a day to assist in the absorption of the extravasation of blood after a fracture so as to reduce the swelling which may take up to 3 to 4 days. Helps to absorb the internal bleeding after a fracture.

Symphytum 6C - More commonly known as comfrey or knitbone or bone set. The name says it all. Promotes fast healing of bones, use with Calc Phos 6X. Take both 3 times daily till better.

The Skin

Bumble Foot

A common affection of the foot pad that can progress into a chronic condition. The cause is from the bacteria Staphylococcus Aureus which is present where ever there are chickens. The bacteria enters the foot through injury.

Symptoms

In maturing birds especially males of the heavy breeds there can be lameness and a reluctance to walk. One or both of the feet may be inflamed, hot, hard and have a pus filled abscess or a dark black scab on the bottom of the foot. Birds may rest on the hocks to keep pressure off the sore.

Postmortem Findings - Pus or cheesy material in foot pad, sometimes hock joints filled with greyish white fluid.

Herbal Treatment

Abscesses are typically caused by a bacterial infection usually starting in a skin break or wound. The first stage is characterized by a painful red swelling after which pus begins to form; this will sometimes discharge itself in a few days. Do not squeeze as this usually causes internal damage and a spread of the wound and infection. Always clean all wounds with a lotion of Calendula or HyperCal which is the tinctures of St John's Wort and Calendula mixed together.

Hot poultices are very effective at drawing the core out of boils and abscesses so here we shall use a hot poultice of slippery elm (half a tea spoon full) with about 4 to 8 drops of castor oil which is also good at drawing out unwanted matter and mix this with a bit of boiling water to form a hot paste. Apply to the area and leave on for 20 minutes and repeat several times till suppuration occurs. After suppuration you can mix together a bit of Calendula and Comfrey creams and apply them to the area. These two herbs working together will speed up the healing time, disinfect and reduce or prevent scaring. Internally give Echinacea for 2 weeks along with Garlic and Burdock for its blood cleansing action.

Homoeopathic Treatment
Remedies with leading symptoms

Hepar Sulph 6C - To ripen a slow forming boil or abscess.

Silica - For more advanced boils or abscesses to encourage them to discharge, for foul smelling discharges or incomplete discharges.

Tarantula Cubenis - For painful hard feeling boils that develop rapidly after a slow start especially

on the back of the neck or on boils where the skin turns red blue or purple. Give this remedy 3 or 4 times daily.

Breast Blister

Also known as Keel Bursitis. The cause is irritation and inflammation due to pressure of the breast bone against roost or floor. Occurs in birds with weak legs or poor feather development offering no breast protection. Most likely where floor is wire or roosts have sharp corners or the litter is wet and hard packed.

Symptoms

In growing or mature Cocks especially of the heavy breed there is a large blister on the keel of the breast. This may sometimes get infected and cause complications.

Resembles - Infectious Synovitis except an uninfected blister is filled with clear or bloody fluid while infected blisters contain creamy or cheesy material.

Prevention - Wrap roosts in something soft to cushion the breast bone or do no provide a roost for Cocks. Allow lots of time free range and cushion bed.

Herbal Treatment

First of all take the prevention measures. The blister can be cleaned with a lotion of Calendula and then lanced and drained of fluid taking note of the color of the fluid and any inflammation in the area. Clean the area again with lotion and then apply Calendula cream. Keep using Calendula until healed. Garlic could be given internally to prevent infection or fight it if present. Keep area clean while healing. If infected use the Homoeopathic remedies Hepar Sulph and Silca as mentioned in Bumble Foot and add St John's Wort to Calendula so you are using a Hypercal lotion.

Scaly Leg

The Scaly Leg Mite Knemidocoptes Mutans is a pale gray round tiny creature that is more likely to attack older birds but also attacks the young if kept with the old. It burrows into the unfeathered parts of the skin raising the scales. The mite spends its entire life on the chicken and is hard to get rid of. Mites slowly travel from bird to bird transmission can be slowed by brushing the perches and chickens legs with a mixture of one part kerosene and 2 parts linseed oil.

Symptoms

Raised scales on the legs, legs thicken and crust over. In severe infestations the combs and wattles are attacked as well as the legs.

Herbal Treatment

For this condition Juliette de Bairacli Levy says the legs should be well scrubbed with soapy water to which a little ammonia has been added then a strong solution of Garlic Brew with a pinch of cayenne pepper with a equal part of vinegar should be rubbed well in twice daily.

The following is a method used by Mrs N Cleary. Make a mixture of one teaspoonful of pyrethrum, 10 drops of Tea Tree Oil and half a teaspoonful of Neem Oil in one litre of water. Dip the legs in the mixture and spray underneath and on their roosts when going to bed. Repeat for a few days. You can also use 1 litre of Neem Leaf Tea with 10 drops of Tea Tree Oil in it for the same effect. Garlic used often is a good preventive for all parasites.

Homoeopathic Treatment - Think of Sulphur 6C or Thuja.

Dry Pox or Fowl Pox

Common in some areas, especially in confined flocks in cold weather. The incubation period is 4 to 14 days and the disease spreads slowly except when being spread by mosquitoes, it can last 3 to 5 weeks in individual birds. There may be a mortality rate of 1 to 2%. The cause is from the Pox Virus that affects a wide variety of birds and survives for many months on feathers and scabs.

Symptoms

In birds of all ages there is a raised clear or whitish wart like bumps on the comb and wattles that grow larger, turning yellowish, and later become reddish brown. Grey or black bleeding scabs appearing singly, in clusters or clumping together, scabs fall off to form smooth scars and sometimes the scabs can spread to the eyelids or other unfeathered areas of the head or neck, vent or legs. There may be decreased growth and egg production.

Herbal Treatment

As this is a viral disease think of Shitake for its antiviral action and use Echinacea for 2 weeks. Garlic applied internally and externally as a lotion on the affected areas. Fast for one day and then follow with a laxative diet. Other herbs to look at are Chickweed to be used internally and externally and Thuja externally (for wart like growths) also think of Calendula externally. After a cure all poultry must be moved and the area disinfected. You could medicate some cream with tincture and use creams on the sores. Add a desert spoon full of tincture to your average size cream jar of Vitamin E cream. Stir until well blended which can take some time.

Homoeopathic Treatment

Although this disease is fairly mild the use of the following remedies may cut short the infective process and prevent secondary infections.

Antimonium Crud 6C - This remedy is associated with typical papular and pustular skin lesions especially with a generally dry skin. Signs of indigestion may be present. Dose 3 time daily for 3 days.

Cuprum Aceticum 6C - A leading remedy for pox like eruptions frequently accompanied by cramps and spasms of groups of muscles. Diarrhea may also be present. Dose 3 times daily for 3 days.

Kali Bich 30C - The pustules assume a crater like form with yellowish discharge. Dose 2 times daily for 5 days.

Variolinum 30C and Vaccinium 200C - Either of these nosodes will be found of values either by themselves or used in conjunction with the mentioned remedies. Dose daily for 3 days.

Thuja 30 - Warts and herpes like eruptions, warty growths that tend to bleed easily.

Excessive Moulting

When moulting becomes so excessive as to expose large areas of bare inflamed flesh on the rumps and throats etc. it is often due to a lack of protein or a acute vitamin deficiency.

Feathers are 85% protein so protein requirements increase during moulting. When your flock is about to moult as indicated by the plumage taking on a dull look begin tossing in a handful of dry cat food into the yard every other day and continue until moult is finished. Only use the dried cat food because it is higher in protein. General symptoms of protein deficiency are slow growth, weight loss, decreased laying and smaller eggs. Excess protein causes Gout.

Herbal Treatment

All the aromatic herbs such as Dill, Anise and Fennel taken internally are god for plumage growth and especially good is all the seaweed family Kelp, Bladderwrack and Dulse. Other good herbs are Nettles, Cleavers and Garlic. Externally you can rub on a lotion of a brew of 2 parts Burdock root with 1 part Castor Oil. Rosemary brew with 2 tablespoons of vinegar to the pint is also good externally. Excessive moulting can also be caused by a unnatural confined life where the bird pulls the feathers out in boredom.

Homoeopathic Treatment

Calc Phos 6C - This tissue Salt ensures the animal makes the most of its nutrition. This is a very useful remedy for the younger animal in the growing stage as it exerts a profound influence on the development of bone and muscle. More suitable for lean animals.

The Reproductive System

Egg Bound

Sometimes eggs get stuck. The egg may be too large or a disease may have caused swelling or paralysed the muscles. The stuck egg then causes future eggs to accumulate behind it distending the Hens abdomen. Unless you can get things moving again the hen will die. Lubricate a fore finger with mineral oil or KY jelly and insert it into the vent. With your other hand push gently on the hens abdomen to force the egg towards the vent. If you can see the egg but it is too big to pass, puncture the shell and remove it in pieces being careful not to injure the Hen. If the egg was stuck in the cloaca to long cloacal tissue may protrude through the vent in which case isolate the Hen to protect her from cannibalism until she returns to normal. Sometimes this condition can be caused by a Calcium and Phosphorus deficiency.

Symptoms

The abdomen becomes very distended and blown looking. The Hen often adopts a peculiar squatting posture with the vent upon the ground.

Herbal Treatment

For this Juliette de Bairacli Levy says the condition can be caused through glandular deficiency and the best safeguard is a daily dose of seaweed and plenty of free exercise. Feed also chopped up Cleavers. For treatment give a dose of Castor Oil with a pinch of Ginger in it and wait 10 minutes and if nothing happens then move onto the next stage by injecting olive oil into the vent, then apply hot cloths and after several minutes try to manipulate the blocking egg with the finger tips. If having problems break up the egg to help removal.

Homoeopathic Treatment

Calc Phos 6C - This Tissue Salt ensures the animal makes the most of its nutrition. This is a very useful remedy for the younger animal in the growing stage as it exerts a profound influence on the development of bone and muscle. More suitable for lean animals.

Dropped Vent (Prolapse)

May also be called a Blow Out. In this condition the lower part of the Hens oviduct turns inside out and protrudes through the vent. Prolapse occurs most often when a Hen starts laying at a to young age, is to fat or lays unusually large eggs. Caught in time the prolapse can sometimes be reversed by applying Hemorrhoidal cream (usually Astringents such as Witch Hazel) and isolating the Hen so as to prevent cannibalism until she improves. This also has been listed as a Calcium and Phosphorus deficiency. Other causes may be being egg bound, diseases of the reproductive system, degeneration of the muscular system and age.

Symptoms

Area of the vent protruding and hanging.

Herbal Treatment

Massage with grease the protruding organ and then carefully press back into position. Place a pad of cotton wool soaked in the astringent and muscle toning Witch Hazel and then lightly bind. Fast for one day and then feed a very light diet entirely of greens, bran mash, molasses, and butter milk. During this treatment stop feeding seaweed as egg laying is not to be encouraged until the condition is better.

Homoeopathic Treatment

Calc Phos 6C - This Tissue Salt ensures the animal makes the most of its nutrition. This is a very useful remedy for the younger animal in the growing stage as it exerts a profound influence on the development of bone and muscle. More suitable for lean animals.

Calc Flur 6C - This is the Tissue Salt specific for loss of elasticity in the tissues and we are looking at prolapse being a deficiency in this.

Sepia 12C - Portal congestion and stasis, tenderness around pelvic area, prolapse.

Tumors

Tumors occur in the reproductive organs of Hens more than in any other animal and are a common cause of poor laying. Old Hens can be prone to slow growing tumors and there is very little information on this as commercial growers don't let their flocks get that old and all the research is put into the young.

Herbal Treatment

Study up on the Herbs Burdock which has a anti-tumor action and the Herb Cleavers which is a good lymphatic cleanser which should help move the rubbish out of the body. Both of these herbs are good blood cleansers. Another two Herbs that can be helpful here are the Shitake and Reshi Mushroom which both have a anti-tumor action but would be more suitable for lowered immunity in this condition.

Salpingitis - Inflammation of the Oviduct

This can be a very common cause of death in layers and usually results from a respiratory infection in which bacteria invades the oviduct via one of the abdominal air sacks. Enteric Bacteria can also be a cause. This seems to be more a opportunist infection so we must really concentrate on attacking hard the beginnings of all disease. Always give Garlic with Echinacea and when Echinacea's 2 weeks are up and things still aren't looking good think about replacing it with Astragalus, Reshi or Shitake. After you think you have won the battle always consider finishing off the job with Burdock cleanse just to be on the safe side.

Turkeys

Turkeys have higher blood pressure than any other fowl so care must be taken that they are not chased as they can suffer a heart attack easily particularly the heavier stags. You can drive them slowly as there flock instinct is strong.

Aspergillosis

Also known as Brooder Pneumonia and Mycotic Pneumonia. This is fairly rare and requires the right circumstances to begin. This condition mainly affects the respiratory condition and sometimes spreads to the liver and brain. The incubation period can be up to 2 weeks and the disease can be acute or chronic. The cause of this disease is from spores of fungus named Aspergillus Fumigatus mixed with other moulds found in the poultry environment. Transmission can be from infected egg shells and contaminated air, food or litter. Sanitation and attention to contaminated eggs may reduce transmission also try to reduce dampness and any other conditions favourable to mould and fungus.

Symptoms

Usually a disease that affects young birds. In chicks under 3 weeks of age there may be gasping, sleepiness, swollen eyes, yellow cheesy material in the eye, loss of appetite, sometimes a nasal discharge, diarrhea, twisted neck, paralysis, convulsions and death. There may be a 10% death rate of those infected and the transmission rate can be high.

In the chronic form in mature birds there may be gasping, coughing, bluish comb, loss of appetite and a rapid weight loss. Only a few birds at a time seem to get infected.

Postmortem Findings - Grayish yellow lungs. In the chronic form in mature birds there may be numerous small yellow to cream colored pearl shaped cheesy nodules in the lungs with the nodules turning green and fury in the advanced stage. There may be circular yellow dished out nodules attached to the air sacs in the chest and abdomen.

Resembles - Infectious bronchitis, Infectious Laryngotracheitis and Newcastle's disease.

Herbal Treatment

Always try to remove the cause so here we should start by evacuating and separating the sick from the healthy and then a decontamination of the living area. Use Echinacea for 2 weeks to build up the immune system. Garlic as usual is our main herb for it is antifungal and exits the body via the mucous membranes and in this case our Garlic will be working in the lungs and air sacs doing its job as it exits. Burdock should be used with the Garlic as it also has a antifungal action as well as its normal use as a blood cleanser and restorative. Some antifungal herbs are Echinacea, Chamomile, Thyme and Sage.

Homoeopathic Treatment

Use Potencies 6C to 30C

Aconitum - Always give at the first signs of a respiratory problem and you may stop the disease from progressing. Eyes red and inflamed with swollen lids, watering. Running nose and sneezing. There may be fever and thirst and usually there is restlessness and anxiety.

Arsenicum - Discharge is acrid, swollen eyelids with tears, chest wheezy, thirst for small quantities, restless, irritable, worse after midnight, Dose every 2 hours for 4 doses.

Allium Cepa 6C - Discharge bland and watery, eyes red and watery and showing photophobia, dose hourly for 4 doses.

Mercurius Sol - Much sneezing, nostrils raw with yellow greenish foul smelling discharge. Swollen eyelids with discharge.

Dulcamara - Sneezing is severe and eyes and nose are generally streaming, there can be a loose cough, the condition is usually caught from the wet and cold. Alternates well with Hepar Sulph.

Blackhead

Also called Histomoniasis and Infectious Hepatitis. This condition is one of the risks of keeping turkeys and chickens together though Mareks disease could even this out. This is rare in chickens but common in turkeys. The areas affected are the liver and ceca. The disease has a incubation period of 7 to 12 days and can be either acute or chronic. The cause is a protozoan infection named Histomonas Meleagridis that is present where ever poultry are except where the soil is dry, loose and sandy, free living forms do not live for long but may survive for years in cecal worm eggs and tend to effect turkeys more the chickens. Transmission occurs from eating infected droppings or protozoa attached to flies, earth worms, grasshoppers, crickets etc. Wild birds spread the condition. Good sanitation and regular worming is good prevention for this condition.

Symptoms

In young birds 4 to 6 weeks old no symptoms or droopiness, drowsiness, weakness, ruffled feathers, increased thirst, loss of appetite, weight loss, darkened face, brownish colored foamy droppings, and sometimes a bloody cecal discharge. The infection rate can be 25 to 50% with mortality up to 30%, the disease peaks at 17 days and subsides by the 28 day.

Post-mortem Findings - Thickened ceca filled with greyish yellow cheesy sometimes blood tinged material adhering to the lining. Sometimes the liver is mottled with circular dished out spots dark at the center and greyish white or yellowish green at the rim.

Resembles - Cecal coccidiosis, Salmonellosis.

Herbal Treatment

With liver problems the best way to start would be a fast so as to rest the liver and give it a chance to sort itself out. Give Echinacea for 2 weeks to build up the immune systems army and also Garlic to start on the battle with the causative protozoan agents. Dandelion and Milk Thistle are two good herbs to look at for serious liver problems. Astragalus can be given after Echinacea's time is up. Treat the diarrhea especially if it is blood with Slippery Elm, if there is lack of appetite mix the Slippery Elm with honey and water.

Homoeopathic Treatment

This will depend on the overall symptom picture but there are certain remedies that have a action on the liver and they include the following.

Aconite 30C - Give at the onset of the problem especially if it arises from cold or there is fever.

Chelidonium 6C - General lethargy yellowish tongue and discoloration of visible mucous membranes, eyes may be weepy, signs of stiffness or pain may be evident over the right shoulder region , stools are clay colored, touch and movement aggravate. Strong yellow discoloration of visible mucous membranes.

Aesculus 30C - Jaundice, the portal circulation becomes congested leading to signs of abdominal discomfort soon after eating, tenderness over the liver, stools are large and hard and the urine becomes discolored, there may be accompanying respiratory symptoms such as coughing up mucous.

Chamomilla 30C - Useful if there is general yellowness of the skin, restless, lying down and quickly getting up.

Lycopodium - A prominent liver remedy, inability to eat much at any one time, very little food appears to satisfy, all symptoms aggravated in the late afternoon and early evening, a good remedy for the old and for lean animals, stools are generally hard.

Mag Mur 30C - Enlargement of liver, jaundice and abdominal pain pronounced. Dose night and morning for 4 days.

China 30C - Weakness and debility, abdominal pain, stools yellow and fluid, increasing weakness. Dose every 3 hours for 4 doses.

Berberis Vulgaris 30C - Sluggish liver conditions with tenderness over lumber region. Skin yellowish, diarrhea symptoms present. Dose 3 times daily for 3 days.

Coccidiosis

See main index

Fowl Cholera

See main index

Fowl Pox - Wet and Dry

See main index

Infectious Sinusitis or Micoplasma Gallisepticum

See Chronic Respiratory Disease in the main index.

Newcastle Disease

See main index

Paratyphoid

See main index

Pullorum

See main index

Staphylococcic Arthritis

See main index

Ducks and Geese

Ducks and Geese are fairly hardy creatures and usually remain healthy through out there life's if parasites and nutrition are monitored carefully. Another advantage they have is that they normally don't live in crowded and confined areas that diseases seem to prefer. Geese and ducks can suffer from most of the diseases mentioned in the book so far so refer to the disease or the system effected. If unsure always treat with Garlic and Echinacea.

Herbal Dosage

Dried Herbs

Dried Herbs are fairly cheap and easy to find and most Health Shops will order in what you need. Dried Herbs can be mixed in the daily ration at a dosage rate of 5 to 20mg per kg of body weight with young and sick animals given the lower dosage. A example of dosage is normally 25 to 40mg per hen per day where they are eating about 125gms a day. Remember mixtures must be adjusted to body weight.

Liquid Herbs

I believe this is the best way of getting most of the herb into the system in the shortest possible time. Liquid dosage can be administered by dosing the drinking water in which case it is best not to do this on hot days as they may go off their water for a while but in a few days they get used to it. Other methods are to make a herbal tea or brew or use Herbal Tinctures that are more concentrated but with these they are usually 50% alcohol so add hot water to the tincture which should evaporate the alcohol.

Dosage Rates - Results have been achieved using 4 to 5mls of **Tincture** to 10 litres of water. This would be good for preventive or tonic treatment.

Herbal Teas - Use 30 grams of fresh herbs or 5 grams of dried herbs to which is added 2 cups of boiling water. Cover so as not to let the essential oils escape and allow to cool. 1 cup of this can be added to the 10 litres of water as above instead of the tincture.

In Acute Situations 10 times the dose is needed especially of Echinacea and Garlic.

These are just suggested doses, when trouble comes separate the sick from the healthy start with the Echinacea and Garlic for in doing this you are covering all bases because you are boosting the immunes system and using a anti biotic, antiviral, antifungal and a wormer all at once. Another reason for separating the sick is so you can observe the droppings and temperature and anything else different from normal which give you additional clues to what is happening and makes it a lot easier if you are going to use Homoeopathic Remedies. Dosage is really observation and common sense.

Homoeopathic Dosage

As a general rule low potencies can be used often (6C to 12C) with an example being really serious cases every 10 minutes while the 30C potencies are used 3 to 4 times a day. Remember once the remedy start to work stop giving it and allow it to do its work. Read the second to last paragraph of the foreword to reacquaint yourself with how Homoeopathic Remedies work.

Last Resorts

Sometimes warm honey and water half and half can revive ailing poultry and warm sweet red wine has been used also. The Homoeopathic Remedy Carbo Veg 6C is known in Homoeopathic Circles as The Corpse Restorer after the fine work it performed hundreds of years ago in the plagues of Europe. Add Carbo Veg to either of the above or as a last resort use all together.

Disease Fighting Herbs

Use Homoeopathic Aconite First in any severe disease that comes on fast as this remedy can sometimes abort the condition, and while this remedy is working you can get your Herbs ready. Echinacea and Garlic are our main herbs and most of the time we start with them at the beginning of a disease especially if we don't know what it is. Always try to focus on the cause as well as the end results so if the cause is bacterial then focus on antibacterial Herbs, if it's a virus focus on antiviral Herbs etc.

Echinacea

Actions - Immune stimulant, anti-microbial, anti-inflammatory, alterative, healing.

Is a infection fighter active against strep bacteria (abscesses and boils), a blood cleanser, (blood poisons, snake bites, poisonous insects) and a glandular and lymphatic system cleanser. Use it particularly for respiration infections and for any disease above the waist. Boosts the white blood cells by stimulating the bone marrow to increase their production.

Uses - All infections, depressed immune function, inflammatory conditions, allergies, effective against both bacteria and viruses. Mostly to fight acute diseases.

Warning - Do not use continually as you will burn out the immune system, for chickens because of their faster metabolism use no longer than 3 weeks but start with a reasonably strong dose.

Garlic

Actions - Immune stimulant, anti-bacterial, anti-viral, anti-protozoan, anti-septic, anti-oxidant, diaphoretic, cholagogue, hypotensive, anti-spasmodic, vermifuge and many more.

The plant is rich in volatile oil and sulphur and because of its remarkable penetrating, disinfecting and mucous expelling powers garlic is a valuable basic remedy for the treatment of all ailments in which the cleansing of the blood stream and expulsion of mucous accumulations is required. Garlic is extremely effective in dissolving and cleansing cholesterol from the blood stream, it stimulates the digestive tract, kills worms, parasites and harmful bacteria, normalizes blood pressure, reduces fever, gas and cramps. Garlic leaves the body via the mucous membranes, so as it is leaving its main actions as a herb are taking place with the one we are counting on being Antibiotic. Garlic is very high in sulphur so think of it as working as a Sulphur antibiotic. Now imagine what we are doing. To prove to you how good this action is take a Garlic oil capsule and put it on the ground, next take off your sock and crush it with your heel and in a few moments you will be able to taste the Garlic exiting the mucous membranes in your mouth.

Uses- All infections, coughs, colds, flu, bronchitis, all fevers, pulmonary conditions, gastric and skin complaints, rheumatism, all worms and also liver fluke, mange, ringworm, ticks and lice.

Externally you can use garlic for ring worm and ear ache, to disinfect wounds and sores, parasitical infections.

Astragalus

Actions - Immune-modulator, anti-viral, adaptogen, hypotensive, immune stimulant, adrenal tonic, diuretic, vasodilator, blood tonic.

Stimulates the natural production of interferon and intensifies the white cell destruction of germs.

A good tonic for strengthening the resistance to disease. Is very useful for animals in a state of chronic debility and fatigue by restoring the immune function. Use as a lung tonic to help expel toxins and pus in flu's, colds and sinusitis. Increases stamina and can accelerate wound healing.

Uses - Boosting immune system, disease preventative, fatigue, healing wounds.

Reshi Mushroom

Actions - Immune stimulant, antibacterial, anti-tumor, adaptogen, rejuvenative, anti-inflammatory

As a immune stimulant it helps to activate the phagocytosis of macrophages and may increase interferon. Aids in the prevention of illness as well as in recovery. Helps normalize blood pressure reduces cholesterol and can inhibit histamine release. Inhibits the inflammation associated with allergies, bronchitis, conjunctivitis and rheumatism. Good for treating chronic hepatitis. Good for over overcoming fatigue, anxiety and stress while improving stamina at the same time.

Uses - Good as a all-round immune booster and restorative tonic. Works well with its fellow mushroom Shitake as they tend to complement each other's actions and together they can be used to attack acute viral diseases. In chronic disease use 1/10 of the recommended dose.

Shitake Mushroom

Actions - Immune stimulant, antiviral, rejuvinative, aphrodisiac.
Animal studies have shown a antiviral and anti-tumor activity as well as the stimulation of killer T cells. Shitake enhances the stem cells in the bone marrow to create more B and T cells. Lowers blood pressure by helping the body get rid of excessive salt and can be used in AIDs like diseases. Stimulates the production of interferon and provides significant protection against type A Virus which causes epidemic influenza.

Uses - Good as a all-round immune booster and restorative tonic. Works well with its fellow mushroom Reshi as they tend to complement each other's actions and together they can be used to attack acute viral diseases. In chronic disease use 1/10 of the recommended dose.

Goldenseal

Actions - Astringent, anti-catarrhal, cholagogue, anti-inflammatory, antibiotic, antiviral, alterative, bitter, laxative, tonic especially for the Digestive System, oxytocic.
Effective anti-catarrhal for drying up mucous membranes, has a activity against Staf, Strep, Chlamydia, Diphtheria, Protozoa, Coccidiosis, E Coli, Salmonella, Cholera and Candida. It is a liver cleanser and antiseptic and is used for internal bleeding and bowel diseases. It lowers blood sugar and is natural insulin.

Uses - Cholera, catarrh, dysentery, gastritis, Giardia, hepatitis, jaundice, TB, malaria, Thrush

Warnings - Avoid during pregnancy, long term use kills friendly bacteria in the intestines and reduces the assimilation of the B Vitamins, avoid in high blood pressure, for short term use only.
Not recommended for laying hens for more than a few does.

Burdock Root

Actions - Alterative, diuretic, bitter, antibacterial, antifungal, anti-tumor.

Animals will not graze this herb with the exception of the ass, but the sliced and bruised roots are one of the finest blood cleansers known to herbalists. The bruised leaves applied externally are a remedy for ring worm and scabies. Soothing to the kidneys and a excellent diuretic.

Uses - Remedy for all blood disorders, rheumatism, skin parasites, skin conditions resulting in dry scaly skin, psoriasis, eczema, dandruff, chicken pox, aids digestion and appetite, aids kidney function and helps with cystitis, speeds up the healing of wounds and ulcers.

Herbal Actions

Anti-biotic - Echinacea, Garlic, Goldenseal, Burdock, Tea Tree Oil. Reshi, Plantain, Rosemary, Neem, Barberry.

Anti-viral - Echinacea, Garlic, St John's Wort, shitake, Goldenseal, Astragalus, Neem.

Anti-fungal - Burdock, Calendula, Goldenseal, Neem

Anti-microbial - Helps the body destroy or resist pathogenic micro-organisms.

Herbs - Cayenne, Echinacea, Garlic, Gentian, Calendula, Plantain, Rosemary, Rue, Sage, Thyme, Wormwood.

Anthelmintic - Destroys or expels worms from the digestive system.

Herbs - Garlic, Gentian, Wormwood, Thyme.

Never mix more than 5 herbs together or you will lose track of what's doing what, if the animal is already on Medication try to find out if there will be any interactions with the medicine and finally to much is not better !. Teas are fairly safe and if you are using tinctures remember that they are about 50% alcohol and cats and some other animals do not like alcohol.

Homoeopathic are safe and easy medicines to use and are effective on animals.

Herbal

Alfalfa

Known also as Lucerne. Rich in nitrates and vitamins is a good tonic food and a kidney cleanser. Excellent for all animals and poultry. Fodder, tonic, nervine, aids in healing allergies, arthritis, morning sickness, peptic ulcers, stomach ailments and bad breath, removes poisons from the body, neutralizes acids, is a excellent blood purifier and thinner, improves appetite and aids in the assimilation of protein, calcium and other nutrients.

Astragalus

Actions - Immune-modulator, anti-viral, adaptogen, hypotensive, immune stimulant, adrenal tonic, diuretic, vasodilator, blood tonic.

Stimulates the natural production of interferon and intensifies the white cell destruction of germs. A good tonic for strengthening the resistance to disease. Is very useful for animals in a state of chronic debility and fatigue by restoring the immune function. Use as a lung tonic to help expel toxins and pus in flu's, colds and sinusitis. Increases stamina and can accelerate wound healing.

Uses - Boosting immune system, disease preventative, fatigue, healing wounds.

Barberry

Actions - Cholagogue, hepatic, bitter tonic, laxative, alterative, antibacterial.

One of the best remedies for correcting liver function and promoting the flow of bile. Indicated for gallstones or jaundice. As a bitter tonic with mild laxative effects it can be used to strengthen and cleanse the digestive system. Acts against malaria and some protozoa eg Coccidiosis. Safe for intermittent or short term use.

Uses - Liver and digestive problems, Coccidiosis, bacterial digestive infections.

Burdock Root

Actions - Alterative, diuretic, bitter, antibacterial, antifungal, anti tumor. Animals will not graze this herb with the exception of the ass, but the sliced and bruised roots are one of the finest blood cleansers known to herbalists. The bruised leaves applied externally are a remedy for ring worm and scabies. Soothing to the kidneys and a excellent diuretic.

Uses - Remedy for all blood disorders, rheumatism, skin parasites, skin conditions resulting in dry scaly skin, psoriasis, eczema, dandruff, chicken pox, aids digestion and appetite, aids kidney function and helps with cystitis, speeds up the healing of wounds and ulcers.

Cleavers

Actions - Alterative, diuretic, anti-inflammatory, astringent, tonic, neoplastic, diaphoretic.

A lymphatic tonic with alterative and diuretic actions which can be used in a wide range of problems where the lymphatic system is involved. The plant is very rich in minerals and silica, gives good strong texture to the hair of animals and the shells of eggs. All animals eat it and poultry especially seek it hence its popular name of goose grass. Good for skin ailments.

Uses - Tonic, eczema, abscesses and tumors, cancerous growths, swollen glands, tonsillitis, psoriasis, cystitis.

Chamomile

Actions   -

Carminative,sedative,antispasmodic,antinflammatory,analgesic,anti septic, antifungal.

It is a famed blood cleanser and pain reducer, reduces tumors (poultice), remedy for female ailments, inflamed gums, use for blood and skin disorders, aches and pains, external and internal inflammations, delayed menstruation, acid uterus and all female ailments, cleanser and toner of the digestive tract, expels worms and parasites, improves and helps appetite. Good nerve tonic.

Uses - Indigestion, colic, diarrhea,insomnia, nervous upsets, anxiety, flatulence. Good for anxiety or changes of routine.

Chickweed

Actions - Healing, anti-inflammatory, astringent, emollient, stops itching, alterative, anti-bacterial.

Rich in copper, highly tonic food for the digestive system and a remedy for all stomach ailments, allergies, colon problems, constipation, piles, rheumatism, skin problems, eczema, psoriasis, itching, irritation, cuts and wounds.

Uses - Bronchitis, cough, laryngitis

Couch Grass

Actions - Diuretic, Demulcent, antibacterial,

Used for kidney stones and gravel along with any other infection of the urinary tract, one of the most important herbs for the urinary system.

Uses - Kidney ailments gravel, stones, urinary tract infections, mild laxative, tonic.

Comfrey

Actions - Demulcent, astringent, healing, expectorant, antiseptic.

Once widely cultivated as a fodder plant, sheep and cows eat it greedily, the impressive wound healing powers of comfrey are partially due to allantoin which stimulates cell proliferation and speeds the healing process inside and out.

Uses - Its old name is knit bone and that describes well what it does. Comfrey also guards against scar tissue from developing incorrectly, all internal hemorrhages including uterine, reunion of wound and fractures, internal ulcers, ruptures, pulmonary problems, bronchitis, irritable cough, ulcerative colitis, skin ulcers and varicose veins.

Dandelion

Actions - Diuretic, cholagogue, anti-rheumatic, laxative, tonic

The herb is blood cleansing and tonic, it has an important effect on the hepatic system and is a supreme jaundice curative herb, the leaves strengthen the enamel of the teeth and the white juices dissolves warts, the plant is well grazed by goats, horses will take quantities of the leaves when cut and well mixed with bran, excellent for anemia because it is high in iron, calcium, copper and vitamins, useful in kidney and bladder problems, skin eruptions, sluggish blood flow, weak arteries, all liver complaints, jaundice, constipation, gallbladder problems and rheumatism.

Uses - Liver and pancreas problems, potassium replacement.

Dill

Actions - Carminative, aromatic, antispasmodic, galactagogue, sedative, digestive tonic.

For the treatment of all digestive ailments especially wind with colic, diarrhea and fevers. Leaves are rich in Vitamin C, iron, calcium and potassium. Can be use externally for lice.

Uses - Digestive problems and lice.

Echinacea

Actions - Immune stimulant, anti-microbial, anti-inflammatory, alterative, healing.

Is a infection fighter active against strep bacteria (abscesses and boils), a blood cleanser, (blood poisons, snake bites, poisonous insects) and a glandular and lymphatic system cleanser. Use it particularly for respiration infections and for any disease above the waist. Boosts the white blood cells by stimulating the bone marrow to increase their production.

Uses - All infections, depressed immune function, inflammatory conditions, allergies, effective against both bacteria and viruses. Mostly to fight acute diseases.

Warning - Do not use continually as you will burn out the immune system, for chickens because of their faster metabolism use no longer than 3 weeks but start with a reasonably strong dose.

Fennel

Actions - Carminative, aromatic, anti-spasmodic, stimulant, galactagogue, expectorant.

The herb possesses highly antiseptic and tonic properties. Peasants drive their flocks to feed upon it owing to the abundance of milk that the herb produces and the sweet odor that it imparts upon the milk. (if the animal is not native they can over gorge and poison themselves).

Arabs use fennel poultices to resolve old and hard tumors.

Uses - Gastric ailments, colic, inflammation of the bowels, acute constipation (raw roots daily), fevers, cramps, worms, indigestion, all eye ailments, bronchitis, coughs, muscular and rheumatic pains use the oil.

Fenugreek

Actions - Expectorant, demulcent, tonic, galactagogue alterative, restorative.

The plant possesses highly aromatic seeds having a powerful disinfectant and emollient lubricant properties. The feeding value of these is about equal to linseed. It is one of the great fattening herbs. The perfect sister herb for garlic enhancing all its powers. Very tonic and eagerly sought by all animals. Rich in vitamins and nitrates, calcium and phosphorus. The whole plant is used.

Uses - Treatment for all gastric weaknesses and ailments, nerves and neuralgia, female ailments, allergies, bronchitis, anemia, bruises, colitis, coughs, diabetes, fever, flu, hay fever, headache, migraines, lung problems, sinus congestion, ulcers, reduces inflammation.

Ginger

Actions - Carminative, anti-inflammatory, vasodilator, stimulant, diaphoretic.

Aids in fighting colds, colitis, digestive disorders, wind, increases saliva, is excellent for the circulatory system and helps increase stamina.

Uses- Indigestion, nausea, feverish conditions, dyspepsia, colic, flatulence. The dried root is used to treat diarrhea associated with cold weather and cold and damp conditions especially where there is a drop in body temperature noted by feeling the comb of the bird and the feet. Also useful for fungal infections.

Garlic

Actions - Immune stimulant, anti-bacterial, anti-viral, anti-protozoan, anti-septic, anti-oxidant, diaphoretic, cholagogue, hypotensive, anti-spasmodic, vermifuge and many more.

The plant is rich in volatile oil and sulphur and because of its remarkable penetrating, disinfecting and mucous expelling powers garlic is a valuable basic remedy for the treatment of all ailments in which the cleansing of the blood stream and expulsion of mucous accumulations is required. Garlic is extremely effective in dissolving and cleansing cholesterol from the blood stream, it stimulates the digestive tract, kills worms, parasites and harmful bacteria, normalizes blood pressure, reduces fever, gas and cramps. Garlic leaves the body via the mucous membranes, so as it is leaving its main actions as a herb are taking place with the one we are counting on being Antibiotic. Garlic is very high in sulphur so think of it as working as a Sulphur antibiotic. To prove to you how good this action is take a Garlic oil capsule and put it on the ground, next take off your sock and crush it with your heel and in a few moments you will be able to taste the Garlic exiting the mucous membranes in your mouth.

Uses- All infections, coughs, colds, flu, bronchitis, all fevers, pulmonary conditions, gastric and skin complaints, rheumatism, all worms and also liver fluke, mange, ringworm, ticks and lice.

Externally you can use garlic for ring worm and ear ache, to disinfect wounds and sores, parasitical infections.

Gentian

Actions - Bitter tonic, gastric stimulant, anthelmintic, cholagogue, alterative.

The root is the medicinal part. Gentian is one of the most important tonic herbs being considered the Prince of the Bitters. Quells vomiting when all other herbs fail, promotes the production of saliva, gastric juices and bile, indicated where there is a lack of appetite and sluggishness of the digestive system.

Uses - Treatment of all forms of digestive weakness, vomiting, nervous ailments including hysteria, malaria, to improve the appetite of all poor feeders.

Liquorice

Actions - Expectorant, demulcent, anti-inflammatory, adrenal agent, anti-spasmodic, mild laxative, used in formulas to help assimilation into the system.

The root part is used , possessing unique pectoral and emollient properties, it is also nutritive and slightly laxative, It contains the building blocks of hormones, has a marked effect on the endocrine system, catarrh, bronchitis, coughs, gastric and peptic ulcers, abdominal colic.

Uses - Treatment of cough, inflamed throat, pneumonia, pleurisy, TB, all catarrhal conditions, gallstones, chronic constipation, mild worms in young animals, female infertility, pains of colic.

Milk Thistle

Actions - Cholagogue, galactagogue, demulcent.

This herb is said to rejuvenate the liver, for problems like hepatitis it is used alone at first as it drains the liver probably by its action of stimulating the gallbladder to release bile. Used to increase milk production in mothers and for gallbladder problems. This herb is a excellent protector of the liver from toxins. It can be used long term to protect the liver from damaged feed and polluted water.

Uses - Liver problems, gallbladder problems, hepatitis, slow acting poisons.

Mullein

Actions - Expectorant, demulcent, mild diuretic, mild sedative, vulnerary, anodyne, astringent.

The herb is famed for its powers in pulmonary ailments being much used in lung ailments of cattle, a bone flesh and cartilage builder, aids in healing respiratory ailments, asthma, bronchitis, sinus congestion, soothing to any inflammation and relieves pain, acts to relieve spasms and clears the lungs, tones mucous membranes of the respiratory system, inflammation of the trachea, painful coughs.

Uses - Coughs, pneumonia, bronchitis, pleurisy, TB, asthma, diarrhea, internal bleeding of the lung and bowel. Laryngotracheitis.

Nettles

Actions - Astringent, diuretic, tonic, alterative, respiratory tonic.

One of the richest sources of chlorophyll in the vegetable kingdom, rich in iron, lime, sodium, Vit C, chlorine and contains much protein. Preventative against many ailments, fattener for poultry, fever, cold, hay fever, allergies, eczema, hemorrhage.

Uses - Treatment of wasting diseases, poor appetite, heat diseases, lung disorders, blood impurities, worms.

Externally - Paralysis, rheumatism, arthritis, loss of muscular power.

Neem

Actions - Anti-inflammatory, alterative, antibacterial, antiviral, antifungal, anthelmintic, bitter tonic, immune stimulant.

The name in Sanskrit means curer of all ailments and another name it is called is village pharmacy. Its antibacterial properties are good for Staph and Clostridia, Neem effectively kills lice and is good for topical applications to skin problems.

Oats

Actions - Nerve tonic, anti-depressant, nutritive, demulcent, vulnerary.

Oats are a strength giving cereal low in starch high in mineral content especially potassium, phosphorus, magnesium and calcium and also the B vitamins. Is a nerve tonic and bone builder, nervous debility, nervous exhaustion, general debility, skin conditions.

Uses - As a nutritive food, remedy and cure for rickets, important for strong teeth, hooves, horns, nails and hair.

Parsley

Actions - Diuretic, carminative, emmenagogue, expectorant.

Well-liked by sheep and goats, improves their milk yield and keeps them free from foot ills.

It is a great enricher of the blood being very rich in iron and copper. Nutrient, digestive tract tonic, diuretic, high in potassium minerals and vitamins, bladder and kidney infections, incontinence, blood cleanser, immune builder, tonic for the blood vessels, aids in afterbirth pains, mainly used as a diuretic, carminative and emmenagogue.

Uses - Treatment of all disorders of the kidneys and bladder, gravel, stones, congestion, cystitis, jaundice, obesity, dropsy, worms, rheumatism, sciatica, swellings of the joints, the root can be used for constipation and obstructions of the intestines.

Plantain

Actions - Expectorant, demulcent, astringent, diuretic, alterative, antibacterial, decongestant.

The whole plant yields soothing mucilage similar to linseed, gentle expectorant while soothing sore and inflamed membranes, coughs, bronchitis. Its astringency aids in diarrhea and cystitis where there is bleeding.

Uses - Treatment of dysentery, hemorrhages, internal obstructions and ulcers, fevers.

Externally - Wounds, sores, ulcers and all bites, eye disorders.

Rosemary

Actions - Carminative, aromatic, antispasmodic, nervine, antibacterial, antiseptic, parasiticide.

It imparts a fine fragrance and tonic properties to the milk of goat and sheep which graze it eagerly. The powdered form is used on wounds as a antiseptic, nerve tonic, carminative, insecticide, acts as a circulatory and nerve stimulant, headache.

Uses - Treatment of all ailments of the heart, rheumatism, fits, epilepsy, paralysis, gastritis, diarrhea, dysentery.

Externally - Wounds, falling hair and nervous spasms.

Reshi Mushroom

Actions - Immune stimulant, antibacterial, anti-tumor, adaptogen, rejuvenative, anti-inflammatory

As a immune stimulant it helps to activate the phagocytosis of macrophages and may increase interferon. Aids in the prevention of illness as well as in recovery. Helps normalize blood pressure reduces cholesterol and can inhibit histamine release. Inhibits the inflammation associated with allergies, bronchitis, conjunctivitis and rheumatism. Good for treating chronic hepatitis. Good for over overcoming fatigue, anxiety and stress while improving stamina at the same time.

Uses - Good as a all-round immune booster and restorative tonic. Works well with its fellow mushroom Shitake as they tend to complement each other's actions and together they can be used to attack acute viral diseases. In chronic disease use 1/10 of the recommended dose.

Shitake Mushroom

Actions - Immune stimulant, antiviral, rejuvinative, aphrodisiac. Animal studies have shown a antiviral and anti-tumor activity as well as the stimulation of killer T cells. Shitake enhances the stem cells in the bone marrow to create more B and T cells. Lowers blood pressure by helping the body get rid of excessive salt and can be used in AIDs like diseases. Stimulates the production of interferon and provides significant protection against type A Virus which causes epidemic influenza.

Uses - Good as a all-round immune booster and restorative tonic. Works well with its fellow mushroom Reshi as they tend to complement each other's actions and together they can be used to attack acute viral diseases. In chronic disease use 1/10 of the recommended dose.

Senna Pods

Actions - Cathartic

One of the most important laxatives because it is also a cleanser and restorative of the entire digestive system. The griping tendency is diminished by the addition of powdered ginger. As heat destroy the properties of this herb it should be prepared as a cold water infusion steeping the pods or leaves for a minimum of 4 hours.

Uses - Treatment of constipation.

Dose - Five large senna pods for a average dog, 7 for sheep, 8 for goats 20 for horses and 24 for cows. Soak in cold water for a minimum of 4 hours but preferably 7 hours. A half cup fill of water for 6 pods, 3/4 cup for 10 pods, one and a half cups for 20 and 24. Add a pinch of ginger to 6 to 10 pods and half a teaspoon to 20 to 24. Give the dose last thing at night at least 2 hours after food has been taken.

Slippery Elm Bark Powder

Actions - Demulcent, emollient, nutrient, astringent.

Slippery elm bark provides a nutritious gruel which also possesses remarkable medicinal properties acting as a poultice both internally and externally. A nutrient and food for very old or young or weak. Coats and heals all inflamed tissues internally and externally and is used for the stomach, intestines, ulcers, ulcerative colitis, enteritis, dysentery, constipation and internal bleeding of the digestive tract.

Uses - Treatment of all digestive complaints especially ulcers for which it is a specific, dysentery, all pectoral disorders including TB, lung and bronchial hemorrhage, wasting diseases, rickets, stunted growth.

Shepherds Purse

Actions - Uterine stimulant, astringent, diuretic.

Possesses important astringent properties, all animals like this herb and poultry seek it eagerly, a gentle diuretic, diarrhea, wounds, reduces excessive menstruation.

Uses - Treatment of hemorrhages internal and external, profuse bleeding of deep wounds, kidney ailments, female problems.

Thyme

Actions - Carminative, antimicrobial, antispasmodic, expectorant, astringent, anthelmintic.

Eaten by sheep and goats and is a milk tonic for them, the whole herb is tonic and antiseptic, A favorite Bee herb and should be planted by all apiaries, dyspepsia and sluggish digestion, can be used for digestive or respiratory infections, use as a gargle for laryngitis or tonsillitis, eases sore throats and coughs, bronchitis, whooping cough, asthma, diarrhea.

Uses - Treatment of all digestive complaints including colic, inflammation of the liver, rickets, all pectoral ailments, hysteria, nervousness, sciatica, retention of afterbirth, inflamed or diseased uterus, metritis, worms including hook worm.

Wormwood

Actions - Bitter tonic, carminative, anthelmintic, anti-inflammatory. The foliage is eaten by horses, cows and sheep. Its chief merits are worm expellant (round worm and pinworm) and tonic. A important herb for female ailments, protects against contagious diseases and plagues, insecticide, hair tonic, as a bitter it stimulates the digestive process, fevers, infections.

Uses - Treatment of all worms, failing appetite, gastritis, gastric ulcers, acidity, enteritis, constipation, jaundice, TB, tumor, pneumonia, pleurisy, all female ailments and bladder problems.

Externally - prevention of falling hair, insecticide especially lice, sores, mange, inflammation of the ear, conjunctivitis.

Homeopathic Supplement

Homeopathy has been around now for hundreds of years and unlike most other forms of medicine its rules have not changed and will not for they are based on a essential truth. The main rule is Like cures Like or if we break down the word Homeopathy homo means the same and pathy means disease. As Homoeopathy is a very hard science to learn and as it kind of sits or balances on the border of hard science and metaphysics I will not try to explain to you what it is here as it would probably take a whole book to do this but I will say this, in the UK and a lot of countries in Europe it is on and paid for by the National Health System and anything that can get a politician to open their purse must work. It is said that Homeopathy sits on a three legged stool. What this means is that if a remedy has at least three symptoms in the same strength as the symptoms you are trying to match then that remedy is a potential cure for your condition or if not cure it will offer the condition relief. The more symptoms you can match to the remedy the better the remedy will work for the rule is likes cure likes not vaguely similar cures. Listed below are some common Homoeopathic Remedies and some of the symptoms they cover. The idea is to find one remedy that covers most of your symptoms. To make the remedies as closer a match as we can we ask lots of questions like the ones below and after we gather all the answers we have what is called a good Symptom Picture which we then try to match as accurately as we can to a Remedy. Most Homeopathic Materia Medicas are set out to answer the questions listed below with the mind symptoms being the most important. Questions on time, position and temperature are good for making a choice between to very close remedies. The best Materia Medica for the lay person is Boerickes and you should be able to view this on a few Homeopathic websites.

Symptom Guide Questions

1. Was there a sudden onset of the condition, at what time?
2. What time of the day does the patient feel either better or worse.
3. What is the effect of motion? jarring? walking? running?
4. What is the effect of drinking fluids? warm and or cold drinks?
5. Is the patient thirsty or not at all? sips or gulps?
6. Is the onset from exertion? overeating? weather changes? emotions?
7. Mental emotional state of patient?
8. Better warm room? warm air?
9. Better cool room? cool open air?
10 Are the respirations upper chest movements or in the abdomen?
11 Respirations - dry or wet?
12 Expectoration - watery or stringy mucous, easy or difficult.
13 Is there coughing
14 Position - better or worse from sitting? standing? lying? lying on which side?
15 Along with the condition is there fever? gas? belching? wind?

Modality - The questions above are covering what the Homoeopaths call modalities which basically mean are covering a condition that makes the patient better or worse. I will list the main Modalities below. The Modalities help us to distinguish which remedy is right for the case especially when we have a group that look as though they may all work which is what I am giving you und the disease heading. Using modalities forces you to think what really is going on, is this the nature of the beast or the nature of the disease.

Time - Better or Worse morning, night, weekly, monthly, seasonally etc.

Motion - Better or Worse first movement, rest, exertion, walking, stretching, rising up etc

Temperature - Better or Worse heat, cold, cold air blowing, sudden change etc.

Body Activity - Better or Worse eating, drinking, urinating, defecating, sleep, coughing etc

Weather - - Better or Worse, damp, sunny, foggy, storms, sudden changes etc.

Senses - Better or Worse - touch, pressure, noise, light, odors etc.

Position - Better or Worse lying, standing, sitting, stretched out, doubled up, right side etc.

Mind - Excitement, anger, fear, stress, better busy, nervous all the time etc.

Now read through all the remedies in the Marteria Medica (Homoeopathic Remedy Reference) and you will notice that most of them have Mind or mental symptoms kind of describing the personalities or moods a good example is Nux Vomica, I think we all know a nasty type of individual that this remedy would be suited to and meaning as though the individual is suited to this remedy then the remedy would have a curative action on them but don't expect it to change the nature of the beast. One of the main rules of Homeopathy is the closer the match of the remedy the higher the Potency you use but if you are not used to Homoeopathy just use the 30C potency and remember what I said about the 3 legged stool. Potency is a measure of strength and depth of action.

Remember as mentioned before Homoeopathy sits on a three legged stool. What this means is that if a remedy has at least three symptoms in the same strength as your symptoms then that remedy is a potential cure.

Note - The best prescribing guide for the layman is **Boerickes Materia Medica With Repertory.**

Another good guide is **The Complete Book of Homeopathy by Dr Michael Weiner.**

I always buy my books on Homeopathy from India as they are quarter the price and there is always a wide selection. Put B. Jain Publishers into the google search engine go to their web site and check out these books and I am sure you will be pleased with what you find.

Disease Nosodes

Nosodes are remedies made from disease material mainly from the tissues, discharges, exudates, excretions, suppurations or secretions of a infected being. Simply stated a Nosode is a homeopathic remedy prepared from a pathological specimen. Rabies Nosode, for example starts with the saliva of a rabid dog and is then potentized. Nosodes have many uses and are widely used in homeopathic practice to help limit cases of infectious diseases and to help during the recovery phase of a disease especially the ones that linger and drag on. There are Nosodes for most infectious diseases of animals and humans the use of Nosodes in this way is referred to as isopathy rather than Homoeopathy. They are often used in farm situations, to limit the spread and the effects of infectious diseases. This has especially been used as a vital component of mastitis control on many farms, both organic and conventional. One documented event about Nosodes dates back to Napoleon marching his Legions through Europe and spreading Typhoid in their wake, the towns that had the best cure rates were the ones where the local Homoeopaths used a Nosode of the disease.

Nosodes can be used in the prevention of infectious diseases in the manner of vaccination but they work by a completely different mechanism then from the raising of antibodies that vaccines work by. As yet it is not actually known how they work but they have survived hundreds of years ridicule by producing results and will carry on doing so. The best known study into Nosodes was done by Dr. Christopher Day of England involving 'kennel cough' in a boarding kennel. At the time he was called in, there were 40 dogs in the kennel with 35 that had kennel cough. About half had been vaccinated for this malady. He gave a Nosode to all the animals that were there and all the dogs that came in through the rest of the summer, which was another 214 dogs. He successfully reduced the incidence of kennel cough from over 90% to less than 2%.

Nosodes used for the prevention of diseases are usually given in the 30C potency. A good dosing regime is one dose given night and morning for 3 days followed by one per month for the next 6 months. This generally provides a good level of protection after the first week. A good example of how this can be used is a puppy given the Nosode of Parvovirus at 3 to 4 weeks of age instead of having to wait for 9 weeks for the vaccination, this way the puppy is protected before given the vaccination. Nosodes can have homeopathic therapeutic properties in their own right. Such Nosodes are found in the Homoeopathic Materia Medica and have undergone a proper 'proving'. Examples are Bacillinum, Carcinosinum, Medorrhinum, Psorinum, Tuberculinum.

Dose - Dr. Surjit S. Makker recommends 20ml of remedy mixed with 8 liters of water for 100 birds. This medicated water should be shaken well and put in drinkers accordingly. For individual birds give them 2-3 pellets by mouth and keep them calm.

Materia Medica

Note - All Homeopathic Remedies are given in Potency and not in material Form.

Aconite

Characteristics - Aconite is best used in the first stages of a illness, especially when fear and anxiety are present. Symptoms appear suddenly, without warning and they may be caused by exposure to cold winds or draughts or by a severe fright. Symptoms are a marked restlessness, animal displays extreme anxiety or fear, high fever with a burning skin, extreme sweating and a burning thirst, a hoarse dry painful cough, bright light noises stress and cold worsen the symptoms, rest and quiet relieves the symptoms. The pains of Aconite are unbearable, sharp, shooting, burning pains, tingling and numbness. A remedy for fevers and inflammatory states, use at the first sign of all fevers, shivering with cold sweats, difficult breathing, animal shows desire for large quantities of water, symptoms worse at midnight, symptoms improve in the open air.

Mind - Great fear, anxiety, restlessness, extreme sensitivity to pain, worry, foreboding.

Better - In open air, warmth, rest.

Worse - In the evening and night, particularly before midnight, lying on affected side.

Allium Cepa

Characteristics - Increased secretions from the eyes and nose, like those of the common cold. Frequent sneezing with watery discharge which burns the nose and upper lip, but the eye discharge is bland and doesn't burn (the opposite of Euphrasia). Tickling in the throat with incessant cough (feels as if larynx is split) holds throat when coughing. Being in cool open air relieves the symptoms, eyelids are swollen and red, abdominal tympany with wind, this remedy is indicated in the early stages of most catarrhal conditions, mild forms of cat flu can be cut short if given early.

Better - Cold room (except cough), open air.

Worse - Evening, warm room, odors.

Antimonium Tartaricum - Ant Tart

Characteristics - Is characterized by a loose rattling unproductive cough such as is often herd in cats. Respiration can be very difficult with much gasping. There is usually thirst for little and often. Symptoms are worse in the evening, lying down and in cold damp weather or a warm room. Confined largely to respiratory diseases, abundant bronchial secretions, great rattling of mucous with little expectoration, drowsiness, debility and sweat.

Mind - Drowsy and despondent, fear of being alone, child will not be touched without whining.

Better - Sitting erect, from burping and expectoration.

Worse - Evenings, lying down, damp cold weather.

Apis

Characteristics - Apis is used for various types of swelling and inflammation such as that from animal bites and bites and stings from insects, it is also used for measles, mumps, sore throats, sore red eyes and fever. Apis is a quick acting remedy for inflammations especially those ones with edema and lots of swelling which is its main use. Acute nephritis with scanty and burning urine there may be some blood in the urine. . Symptoms are swelling with edema which makes the effected parts look shiny, red and puffy, the swollen parts feel soggy and waterlogged, a fever that develops rapidly but without thirst, extreme restlessness and fidgeting, an irritable nature and perhaps jealous, cool air and cold compresses relieve the symptoms. Pains are burning and stinging, arthritis with swelling, animals seek cold surface to lie on, swollen eyelids, may be swollen ears, may be blood in the urine, in the horse and cow there may be edema in the lower limbs while in dogs abdominal dropsy is seen. Symptoms get worse from heat and improve in the open air and from cold bathing.

Mind - Apathy, indifference, awkward.

Better - By cold, (room, air or application)

Worse - From warmth, pressure, late in the afternoon, from sleeping.

Arnica

Characteristics - Bruises and similar injuries where the skin is unbroken and there is mental or emotional shock. Symptoms are any type of bruising or similar injury caused by crushing, squeezing or wrenching, muscles strains which feel sore and bruised, shock after accidents, there is a fear of being touched because of the pain, good for the soreness after birth and medical operations.

Arnica can be used in potency and also as a cream. The cream must not be used on broken skin or wounds. Animal shrinks away when you try to touch it, symptoms improve when lying down.

Mind - Fears touch or approach, whole body oversensitive.

Better - Lying down or with head low.

Worse - Least touch, motion, damp and cold.

Arsenic Album

Characteristics - Burning pains relieved by heat, anxious, restless, weak and chilly with an air of fear and hopelessness. Anxiety or restlessness are often present where this remedy is indicated. Discharge from eyes and nose are watery and acrid causing ulceration in those regions. The mouth is usually dry and the patient is usually thirsty. Dramatic vomiting and diarrhea often simultaneously indicate its use if the modalities agree. The patient may have wheezing respiration and allergic asthmatic conditions can respond well. The skin can be dry, scaly and scruffy. Symptoms are worse for cold and wet better for warmth. Tries to find relief in motion but immediately feels weak with movement. Restless, feels cold, complains of general weakness, discharges burn the skin.

Mind - Fear with despair and restlessness.

Better - Warmth, open air, relieved by sweat, hot drinks, lying down (but restless).

Worse - Cold air, after midnight eg 1 to 3am. Wet damp weather and near sea shore.

Belladonna

Characteristics - This is one of the great fever remedies, conditions requiring its use usually being of violent and sudden onset. Heat, redness, pain and swelling characterize its symptoms. It is one of the main remedies used in convulsions. Pupils are usually dilated which is a keynote for this remedy. Acute ear inflammation where there is heat, pain and swelling respond well. The mouth is usually dry and there is great thirst. With Belladonna always think BIRDS. B for burning, I for irritability, R for redness, D for delirium and S for spasms.

Mind - Hallucinations, delirium, rages, bites, strikes, desire to escape.

Better - For quiet, dark, rest with slight warmth.

Worse - For noise, touch or jarring motion.

Bellis Perennis

Characteristics - Trauma to abdomen and pelvic organs especially after surgery and child birth if arnica does not give relief. Injuries to the nerves with intense soreness, back ache from hard physical work such as gardening, pain is bruised sore and aching, better cold presses, worse touch, after getting wet.

The animal is unwilling to move and when made to do so evinces pain, muscular stiffness is prominent.

Worse - Left side and cold wind.

Bryonia

Characteristics - This remedy shows both diarrhea and constipation symptoms, the latter usually in chronic conditions. The mouth is often dry and there is great thirst. The tongue is often coated yellow. It is of great help in many cases of rheumatism or arthritis where the symptoms agree. There is often respiratory signs with a hoarse hacking cough. All symptoms are worse for movement and better for rest.

Mind - Irritable, delirium.

Better - Lying on the painful side, pressure, rest and cold things.

Worse - Warmth, motion, morning, eating and touch.

Calendula

Characteristics - The part used is the Flowers and it is used for wounds and skin irritations, it is healing, soothing, anti-inflammatory, astringent, anti-fungal and anti-microbial.

Use as a lotion for cuts, grazes, infected sores, fungal infections, any skin inflammations, regulates the oil production of the skin so is good for acne, to stop bleeding, for bruises and sprains, skin ulcers and minor burns and scolds.

Note - The tincture of this is used as a lotion diluted at 1 to 10.

Cantharis

Characteristics - Important first aid remedy for minor burns and for other pains that feel burning and fiery, also has a healing effect on the bladder, urethra and other parts of the urinary tract where burning pain is the key symptom, burns and scalds especially where blistering and inflammation occur, sunburn, insect bites that feel hot and burn, cystitis. Pains are violent burning, cutting, stabbing or smarting, rawness, use when the animal appears distressed when passing urine, or tries to pass and cannot. Better from warmth rest and rubbing.

Mind - Furious delirium, acute mania generally of a sexual type, crying, barking.

Better - From rubbing

Worse - From touch or approach, from urinating, from drinking cold water.

Carbo Vegetabilis

Characteristics - Patient exhibits mental and physical sluggishness and symptoms come on slowly, generalized weakness of all functions especially digestion, overweight, torpid, lazy, complaints of coldness, pains usually described as burning, pressing pains, wishes to be fanned, digestive problems such as belching often accompany any illness.

Mind - Aversion to darkness, sudden loss of memory.

Better - Being fanned, passing gas, rest.

Worse - Morning and evening, exertion, cold, tight clothes at abdomen.

Causticum

Characteristics - Burns and burning pains such as cystitis also used for dry coughs, burns to the skin especially with marked inflammation and blistering, coughs, laryngitis and hoarseness from straining and over using voice, cystitis especially with involuntary passing of urine when coughing, chronic cystitis, exposure to cold dry air may make symptoms worse.

Mind - Least thing makes it cry, sad, hopeless. Ailments from long lasting grief.

Better - In damp wet weather, warmth.

Worse - Cold winds.

Euphrasia

Characteristics - Affects the mucous membranes of the eyes, nose and chest producing copious watery secretions, eye secretions cause smarting of the skin while the nose discharge is bland. Used for conjunctivitis, eye strain generally but especially from computers, eyes that feel sore and inflamed and look red, hay fever symptoms including a tickly throat, sneezing, a runny nose, and itchy red watering eyes. Sunlight wind and warmth worsen the symptoms. Use for Dogs who have had their head out of the window for to long, symptoms better in dim light or darkness, in all species a tendency to diarrhea occurs.

Better - In the dark

Worse - From light, indoors, in the evening.

Hypericum

Characteristics - Used for bruises and other injuries especially to nerve rich areas like the fingers, lips, ears, eyes, tail bone, good for the pain of puncture wounds of any cause eg animal or insect. Helps with the pains after operations especially amputations. Pains are violent shooting pains along a nerve path, burning, tingling and numbness. Worse from shock and touch and better from rubbing, horse fly bites, symptoms worse cold better warmth.

Mind - Anxiety, melancholy, effects of shock.

Better - Bending head backward.

Worse - Cold, dampness and touch.

Ipecac

Characteristics - Indicated for complaints of persistent nausea not relieved by vomiting, ailments caused by eating rich or indigestible type of foods such as ice-cream, sweets etc., useful to stop bleeding if blood is bright red.

Mind - Easily irritated, child cries or screams continuously, wanting something but not sure what they desire, holds everything in contempt.

Worse - Warm, moist weather, lying down.

Kali Bichromicum

Characteristics - Has a affinity for the mucous membranes of the body, tough stringy viscid secretions sometimes forming thick yellow green mucous, sinus infections, suited for fleshy fat light complexioned people, general weakness.

Better - Heat

Worse - Cold, beer, morning, undressing.

Kali Carbonicum

Characteristics - Has a affinity for the mucous membranes digestive and respiratory, very tired, anemic, flabby tissues which may be swollen, sweat, backache, weakness, many conditions have a aggravation at 2am to 4am, often stays immobile when ill.

Mind - Very irritable, hypersensitive to pain, despondent.

Better - During the day, sitting down, bending forward, warmth.

Worse - Cold weather, between 2am and 4am.

Lachesis

Characteristics - Many symptoms tend to be left sided, cannot bear tight clothing, symptoms worse on awakening, symptoms relieved with onset of the menstrual flow. Short dry cough, feels relief after coughing up watery phlegm, feeling of constriction in throat and chest, better bending forward.

Mind - Overly talkative, impatient, sad, jealous, no desire to mix with world.

Better - Release of pressure, eating fruit, cold, discharges.

Worse - Pressure, touch, after sleep, heat, hot weather.

Ledum

Characteristics - Has a action on the capillaries and is useful for cleaning up bruises especially around the eyes, mainly used for puncture wounds made by sharp points such as nails and wood splinters and insect bites and stings especially ones that don't heal properly and look blue and puffy. Wounds that feel cold to the touch, septic conditions, sprains, pains are throbbing, tearing , prickling, they shoot upwards, stiff and sore. Better cold, cold bathing. This remedy was used in the past along with hypericum to ward off tetanus especially in deep wounds

Better - From cold.

Worse - At night and from heat.

Lycopodium

Characteristics - Exerts most of its effects on the digestive organs, liver, kidneys and respiratory systems. The patient dislikes being left alone and appears apprehensive. The nose is often blocked and there may be blisters on the tongue. Eating a little food always satisfies the appetite but appetite is very marked. The belly is usually bloated. The stool appears hard and small and is expelled only with difficulty accompanied by ineffectual straining. Urination is also a slow process and the urine has a red sediment. Symptoms are worse for heat generally and better for cold.

Mind - Melancholy, afraid to be alone, apprehensive.

Better - By motion, on getting cold.

Worse - From heat.

Natrum Sulphuricum

Characteristics - A good liver remedy, emotional and mental difficulties arising after head injury, useful in problems associated with rainy weather and dampness, patient feels every change from dry to wet weather, may remove excess water and fluid retention from the body.

Mind - Lively music saddens, melancholy, inability to think, dislikes to speak or be spoken to.

Better - Dry weather and environments, pressure, change of position.

Worse - Damp weather, damp basements, lying on left side.

Nux Vom

Characteristics - The remedy for overindulgence, adapted especially to thin irritable energetic people who attend with great detail to tasks, quarrelsome, nervous, intelligent, hypochondriacal, oversensitive to noise music and light, craves stimulants.

Primarily used in the digestive sphere, its greatest reputation is in helping disturbances following overeating of unsuitable foods. Feces is usually hard but diarrhea can follow overeating. There is abdominal discomfort, flatulence, irritability and sensitivity to noise. Symptoms are generally worse for noise and better after rest or for damp weather.

Mind - Very irritable, sensitive to all impressions, malicious, disposed to reproach others.

Better - Wet weather, lying down, uninterrupted nap.

Worse - Overeating, mental over exertion, sensory stimulation ie sound, sight, touch etc.

Phosphorus

Characteristics - Irritated and inflamed mucous and serous membranes are the key feature of this remedy. Is a very sudden remedy with suddenness of symptoms. The patient is sensitive to loud and sudden noises (eg thunder fireworks etc). Degenerative processes and bone destruction respond well to Phosphorus. Food is suddenly vomited back up when it has been warmed in the stomach, gums can be ulcerated and bloody. Hepatitis, jaundice, pancreatic disease and nephritis come into its sphere. Urine may be bloody. A very painful cough is also a symptom. Wounds that perpetually bleed may also be helped. The patient is usually in poor body condition. Symptoms are worse for touch, exertion, in the evening and during thunder storm. Better for cold and sleep.

Mind - Low spirits, restless, fidgety.

Better - In the dark, lying on the right side, from the cold, sleep.

Worse - Touch, from exertion and in the evening.

Pulsatilla

Characteristics - Often indicated for those with mild, gentle, timid yielding dispositions who are easily moved to laughter and tears, The Pulsatilla person wants to be held and loved, moods changeable and fickle, the patient is chilly but desires strolling in cold air, symptoms are erratic and change frequently, pains are wandering, pains that grow gradually in intensity, fever without thirst despite dry mouth, bland yellow discharges.

Mind - Weeps easily, timid, fears to be alone - dark - ghosts, likes sympathy and fuss, highly emotional, easily discouraged, sensitive.

Better - Open air, cold applications, consolation relieves symptoms.

Worse - Evening before midnight, warmth, after eating fat rich food.

Rhus Tox

Characteristics - Is the most famous of the rheumatic remedies. The skin and muscular skeletal system are its main spheres. Small red papules in the skin and sometimes vesicles are typical lesions with much scratching. In all cases of damage to muscles think of Rhus and the symptoms of arthritis which are worse after rest particularly if this follows strenuous exertion. The symptoms improve with limbering up, The worst pains are seen as the animal arises from its bed.

Mind - Listless, sad, extreme restlessness, great apprehension at night.

Better - Warmth, walking, from stretching out limbs.

Worse - During sleep, cold wet rainy weather and at night.

Ruta

Characteristics - Has effects on the joints, tendons, cartilages, and the periosteum which is a fine membrane that covers bones and gives it that shiny look, it is also used for eye strain where the vision goes dim.

Used for painful bruises affecting the bones, dislocations, strains to the tendons or joints, aching with restlessness, pains are gnawing, digging, burning, bruised, sore as if beaten, bones as if broken, pain deep in the bones, rheumatism.

Better - From lying and warmth.

Worse - From over exertion, touch, cold wet weather.

Silica

Characteristics - Fits the shy chilly patient who is reluctant to enter the room, chronic inflammatory conditions such as sinus, helps in the removal of foreign bodies such as splinters and seeds, ripens abscesses, ailments attended with pus formation. Use silica and be prepared to use it for a while sometimes up to 3 weeks.

Mind - Faint hearted, anxious, yielding.

Better - Warmth, wet or humid weather.

Worse - Morning, from lying down, cold.

Staphysagria

Characteristics - Suits sensitive people who suppress their feelings and suffer in silence or who boil over with indignation, remedy for cuts and wounds especially those that are from medical procedures and have the mentioned feelings. Nervous states of animals. The pains are stinging, stitching, smarting, squeezing, as if stabbed by a knife. Worse from touch, emotions and suppressed anger.

Better - Warmth, rest at night.

Worse - Touch on affected parts, loss of fluids.

Symphytum

Characteristics - Causes bone to grow and promotes fast healing should be given for all fractures. Used for injuries to the hard parts of the body while arnica is for the soft parts. Also used for eye injuries caused from blows.

Caution - Do not use if a pin has been placed in the bone as the pin has to be removed latter.

Tarentula Cubensis

Characteristics - For abscesses, boils, carbuncles, swellings of any kind but especially on the back of the neck where the skin turns black, red/blue or purple with great pain. Deep septic conditions with hardening of the effected part, condition comes on fast, pains are burning, stinging, throbbing, pricking like a needle.

Worse - Night.

Urtica Urens

Characteristics - Can be used for burns and also for cystitis where the urine burns the skin and there is dificulty passing urine. Symptoms are stinging pains, swellings particularly blistery swellings, itching.

Worse - Cool moist air, touch.

Notes

Global Warming Edition
Fire, Heat Stress and Global Warming

As I am writing this during summer in the State of Victoria, Australia in the Countryside, the top of Australia in the Northern Territory has a fire burning which is the size of Spain. It just seems to be getting worse all the time. Australia is notorious for its massive fires and now the severity is getting worse, but luckily over a period of 20 years we have changed our habits and ways of thinking and quite a few times now we have managed to save ourselves when the Authorities were overwhelmed and could not help, or the roads were cut off so they couldn't get there anyway. Most farms big, small or Hobby Farms and even isolated properties now have trailers with a 1000 litre IBC tank hooked up to a pump and hose that can be transported where it is needed. Quite a few times now when the roads are blocked local communities have saved themselves with these trailers and on a lot of occasions some people call their friends for help and to bring their fire trailers over. With mobile phones they have now found that they can organize themselves and get multiple trailers out to deal with spot fires and have the situation under control before the Authorities get there. Now with the technical advancement and the falling of prices for drones you can even have a look at what is happening before you even get there or on your way. As far as I am concerned this is the way it should be and as the situation is only going to continue to get worse more people should start to prepare themselves for the worst. As the conditions get worse across the globe many people in remote areas are going to have to learn to look after themselves for as usual most of the help will go to the cities and large towns, so now is the time to start making your plans.

High Temperature Animal Management
Needs Good Planning

You need to develop a plan for days of high to extreme temperatures to ensure that your animals will have sufficient shade and water when needed in extreme weather conditions. Extreme heat causes significant stress for all animals with some suffering more than others, so now is the time to review your planning and farm infrastructure so as to provide shaded areas with good ventilation to maximise heat loss. As a gauge we will use 36 degrees Celsius as our danger mark especially if the heat is dry, if it is humid we can relax a bit, but it's time to get our act together. Managing animals in high temperatures requires good forward planning and keeping an eye on the weather forecasts along with developing a plan for days of high to extreme temperatures is essential in ensuring that your animals will have sufficient shade and water on those very hot days. More shade and water troughs would be a good start along with checking the animals more frequently during the hottest days at the hottest times of the day for signs of heat stress, along with all the water points to ensure animals have access to plenty of clean cool water. Make sure troughs or containers are firmly fixed so they cannot overturn and are clean, well designed and maintained to prevent injuries. Make sure the stock does not have to walk too far for water and that they know where all the water areas are and if you use large concrete troughs these will to help keep the drinking water cool. Extreme heat causes significant stress for all animals and it's up to you to ensure the welfare of your animals is maintained. Animals need to be checked regularly throughout the day for signs of heat stress. Remember with Global Warming there is no such thing as normal weather patterns anymore and it's going to get worse before it gets better, if it ever gets better, but that's up to our Governments and the rich elite of the world which makes it even more depressing.

Heat Shelters for Animals

Animals need shelter during extended periods of extreme temperatures especially the very young or old and animals that are in poor condition or sick. Every farm is different but they are all going to get hit with Climate Change one way or another along with the country areas and their populations, so now is the time to have a good look around and consider improvements and see what there is that's going to give you problems in the future. Walk around the property and try to see what's going to cause you trouble in the middle of summer. Where do I need to put shade, are there any sheltered areas that you could use or fence off in an emergency and may add more trees and shade. Due to storms getting worse it may be time to have another good look at your high ground and figure out how you could use it in a flood and maybe how you could save the water by creating dams or ponds. About 30 years ago I was on a farm built on the side of a hill in the subtropics in Queensland that had a near hit by a cyclone. We had to wait a week before we could get into town, and even then we had to pile everyone onto a truck to get there as a car would have been washed away. Ten years later I was on a farm in South Australia 60 to 70 kilometres North of Adelaide during a drought and they stopped us from using the slasher on the back of the tractor, as when the slasher hit a rock the spark off the blade would cause a fire. To be honest I am glad my times nearly up as the future is not really looking all that bright and the reality is that it's up to you now to look after and protect you and yours with maybe a little help from your friends. Now let's have a good look at what's out there to keep your animals cool and healthy in the heat to come. **The best type of shelter during extreme heat should protect the animals from the sun and allow for the cooling effect of wind.** Don't forget to put some water close by. Pets and small animals should be moved to cool areas of the house or a shed.

1/. **Shade Sails** - My favourite and the easiest and cheapest to do is the Shade Sails. These are easy to set up and can be used as a large or small scale setup, or just in the places where you need them. The simplest is the sail on three posts. The best ways to use these are to find the areas on your property with a bit of natural shade and see how much you can increase it using a simple cheap sail with 3 posts. A good and natural spot to choose would be where a stream is in a valley where the animals would head to naturally or any other area in your land that has a natural shelter or one that could be made easily. On different farms I have noticed that animals tend to hang out in certain areas when they rest so this may be a good spot. Another advantage is that you can easily take the shade down for winter so it doesn't have to wear out fast. Shade sails are about the fastest, cheapest and easiest way to go and are a good first choice with fast results.

2/. **Trees and Shelter Belts** – Lots of farms have these; usually they are in an area where it was not worth the effort to get rid of them or too hard to access, or even a danger to the livestock. Maybe it's time these areas are re-examined again to see if they can be used fully or partly as a Heat Refuge. While you are doing this also consider where you could place new trees with large canopies that are fast growing and native to you area. Also consider placing one of these trees beside each water trough to slow down the evaporation rate. Shelterbelts or Hedges are a good idea and can be as big and complex as your imagination. Always have them crossing the farm going East to West so when the sun rises in the east the animals can use the shade on the west and the opposite in the afternoon, so that leaves us with only the mid-day sun to sort out. Always remember to leave regular gaps in the belts and hedges so animals can pass through them easily but also more importantly to allow a breeze to blow through the gaps to help cool the animals. Trees have a cooling effect due to absorption of heat by the leaves. Always check out the fodder trees that can be grown or even better are native to your area and always try to make everything multi-purpose. For those that are interested in this and want more information find yourself a Permaculture Manual as that will give you all the information you need along with plants you can use as stock feed and trees you can use as what they call Pioneer Plants, which you use to protect and fertilize the tree you want to grow which dies off latter after it has finished its work.

3/. - Placement and Construction of Livestock Sheds – Placement is the first and most important consideration especially for heat, but saying that if you live in a place where they have nasty cold winters and lots of snow you will have to decide between which is worse for you and plan accordingly. In winter the sun is low on the horizon so maybe think about making a sleeping and resting area on the longest wall of the structure so as to capture the most heat in winter, then in summer when the sun is above it will run along the roof. Aluminium or galvanised steel are ideal roofs for shelters, kennels, and chicken coops as these materials are very good at reflecting the radiative rays of the sun. Other common construction materials are corrugated iron, timber and shade cloth. You may want to consider having the structures east to west so in summer the sun runs across the roof and maybe insulate the east and west walls. **Outdoor poultry houses** should be positioned in shaded areas away from the sun and in a place where it can get good airflow. Use wide overhangs at the eaves and solid end walls so as to make as much shade as possible. Don't forget that an angled roof will reflect more heat at the hottest time of the day and leave you room for adding insulation in the future if things get worse. Place the nesting boxes in the coolest part of the structure or maybe back to back down the centre as this might be a better place for all the seasons. Again consider insulation on the east and west walls. With any farm construction it is always better to build slightly bigger then smaller as you don't want the risk of animals getting crushed, smothered or injured and always consider the entrance and door sizes as again it's better to make them bigger and avoid future problems.

Heat Stress Tolerances for livestock

Animals at high risk of heat stress are the young, black and dark coloured animals and animals that have been housed and not usually out in the sun with fair skin such as pigs. As always the sun will make it worse for the sick and injured of all kinds and greatly increase the rate of water needed. Heat stress tolerances also vary between different species and different places where animals are farmed so we need to know what's happening in our own area, and how it is going to affect the livestock and what the future outlook may be, as there is no going back now. Your area may not be suitable anymore, or another breed of the same species might be happier in your area. Better to make the decisions sooner than later as it will be far cheaper in the long run. In Australia I was on a farm up North in the subtropics so we got Anglo-Nubian Goats who handled the temperature a lot better than us and most of the other animals and as an added bonus we found them to be highly intelligent. Next we will take a look at how heat stress affects our main animals.

Handling Hot Days and Transport Animals

Try to do all the animal work in the cool of the mornings or the evenings. It is not good for you or the animals to work in extreme heat unless absolutely necessary or in an emergency such as a fire. Some of the farms I have worked on in very hot areas we worked from 6am to 10am and then 2pm to 6pm, which made life more bearably for both the human and the animals. For cattle research has shown that movement or handling during hot weather can increase their body temperature by 0.5 to 3.5° C. Increased body temperature or heat stress will cause losses in livestock and impact on their ability to function. Moving animals during cooler hours can decrease the impact of high temperatures, with a good example being a delay in milking by an hour or more in the evenings can result in an increase in production of up to 1.5 litres per day per cow. Transport of animals should be planned so that climatic extremes are avoided and animals are transported during the cooler hours of the day or at night. I know of an example that went really wrong when the driver was doing all the right things, he was carrying chickens from Adelaide to Melbourne which is a distance of 750 kilometres. He was carrying chickens in cages with water on a semi-trailer which they always tarped so as to keep the wind off the chickens, and always drove through the night so there would be no heat stress and always stopped at the half way point to check that everything was fine. In the last part of the trip the tarp ripped on the side close to the back on the trailer and the poor chickens there had to endure 110 Kph winds for a few hours resulting in about a quarter of them were very naked and not happy. Unfortunately the new owner was not very impressed and asked him what the hell did you do to them, which was about the same time as the drivers offsider burst out in hysterical laughter. This was just one of those things, the driver did everything right, he drove in the cool air of night, he only stopped once to check the load and that was just for 5 minutes. The general rules for transporting animals especially sheep and cattle in severe heat conditions are to use the safest and quickest roots, try to do it in one trip so the breeze through the truck keeps the animals cool. If it is necessary to stop, park the vehicle in the shade and at right angles to the wind direction to improve wind flow between animals during hot weather. Keep the duration of stops to a minimum to avoid the build-up of heat while the vehicle is stationary. In extreme heat reduce stocking densities by about 15% so as to encourage more breezes throughout the trailer to keep the animals cool. In some States and especially in the outback you have to have powerful rifles so if you have an accident you can humanly put down those animals that need it.

Heat Stress Effects on Animals

The general signs of heat stress are panting, increased respiration rate, increased water intake, loss of appetite, listlessness or lethargy, increased salivation and in severe cases unconsciousness and the possibility of death. Here we will go through the different animals and see how they handle excessive heat and what we can do to prevent problems. If your animals are showing signs of heat stress you need to cool them down so start with taking them to the shade, with the best areas being were there is a breeze. To add to this you could use a water sprinkler capable of adding a fine misty spray to reduce the heat even further. Do not soak the animals, just a little bit of mist frequently. If animals are too stressed to move, pick them up and move them or provide shade where they are especially for the larger and heavier animals such as cattle. With cattle the easiest solution is to get the truck and use the truck to block the sun then provide water in 20 litre buckets (or whatever you have), encourage them to drink small amounts often as, a large amount may cause shock and death. After that try to find the biggest water mister bottle you can and spray just spray one of them and see how they handle it especially on the legs and feet, don't try to pour a bucket of cold water on them as the shock could be too much, but they may like a big wet towel put over them. **I have decided to start here with Humans because if you don't look after yourself and get it you are not going to be much use to your animals.**

Humans and Heat Stress

If you are have to deal with heat stress in animals then it's time to learn how to treat Humans with the same condition, as you may be the next victim. This condition can sneak up on you without you realizing what is happening especially if the sun is directly on you head. Heat exhaustion is the beginning of the journey towards heat stroke. One of the fastest ways of getting there is wandering around in the sun on a hot sunny day of over 36 degrees Celsius without a hat on in the middle of a cloudless day. This means the sun is right above you and is beginning to cook your brain very fast. You can develop some really weird symptoms fast and need to get out of the sun. Unfortunately I went through this at about 21 and learned my lesson well. Now that the climate is hotter this is a lesson we should all learn especially for our children's sake as they are the ones that are vulnerable now. Start with your basic First Aid. A pre-warning of Heat Stress can be **Heat Cramps** which usually happen when you work outside in the heat and are sweating a lot and you've used up your excess fluid, so the body decides to tell you by starting to cramp.

Signs of heat stress
Excessive sweating and cold, pale, clammy skin.
Headache.
Dizziness and confusion.
Loss of appetite and feeling sick.
Nausea and or vomiting.
Cramps in the arms, legs and stomach.
Fast weak pulse.
Tiredness weakness.
Being thirsty.
Headache.
Fainting.
Decreased Urine Output.

Take this as your warning sign and get rehydrated and have a rest in a shady cool area. Heat cramps are the mildest form of heat related illness. They are painful muscle cramps and spasms caused by your body's loss of salt and fluid due to excessive sweating. Heat cramps can occur during or after intense exercise and can be a symptom of a more serious heat exhaustion. To relieve the cramps drink some water or even better a rehydration solution which should be in every first aid kit and rest in a shaded cooler area and finish the work in a cooler part of the day. Sometimes we can miss out on the cramps and slowly work our way to Heat Exhaustion without releasing till it is too late. Check all the symptoms and start treatment quickly so as to not make the condition worse. The best you can do is get the patient into a cool house with the air-conditioning running and offer them a long cool drink or even better one with a rehydration formula mixed into it and observe the patient and see what happens. Are they over dressed for the conditions? If so suggest to them that they are overdressed for the conditions. If you are worried that the condition is getting worse don't hesitate to call for an ambulance as the phone operators are usually highly trained and can go through the issues with you.

Signs of Heatstroke
Hot, Red, Dry or Damp Skin.
Cessation of sweating.
Body temperature of 38C (104F) or higher.
Fast Strong Pulse.
Decreased urine output.
Rapid and shallow breathing.
Rapid heartbeat.
Elevated or lowered blood pressure.
Confusion and disorientation.
Can be nausea and Dizziness.
Can be seizure.
Fainting - often the first sign in the elderly.

Remove the person from the heat to a cool shady area, if serious especially in the old and young seek emergency help if available. Remove excessive clothing and take note of vital signs such as pulse and temperature and record them along with the worst symptoms. Cool the person with whatever means available but be careful not to shock them, again it's the young and old you have to be very careful with as a shock could be the last straw. Put in a cool tub of water or a cool shower, spray with a garden hose, sponge with cool water, fan while misting with cool water, or place ice packs or cold, wet towels on the person's head, neck, armpits and groin. Was the person just affected by the heat? Or were they working and exerting themselves in the heat? Is it humid weather? Have you been drinking alcohol (dehydration)? When was the last time you had a drink of water? Without a quick response to lower body temperature, heatstroke can cause your brain or other vital organs to swell, possibly resulting in permanent damage which is why this condition is an emergency situation so it is best to get as much information as you can get, especially of any medication they are taking and talk to the emergency services and see what they have to say.

Homoeopathic Remedies For
Heat Stress and Heat Stroke

Below are Homoeopathic Remedies that can be used for Heat Stress and Stroke. These remedies can be used by Humans and Animals. Instead of giving a higher dose when you consider the situation is getting worse it may be better to go to a higher Potency and see what happens. If the situation gets worse which can easily happen in this condition especially in the old and young and you require Ambulance or Medical Treatment, ensure they know the patient has taken Homoeopathic Remedies as the remedies may be masking some of the symptoms. The most important things you can do while waiting medical help is to keep the patient hydrated, cool, comfortable and in a positive mood knowing that help is on the way.

Remedies Heat Exhaustion

China 6C to 30C - Feeling totally wiped out, drained with trembling. Very useful where there has been excessive sweating and severe dehydration is a factor.

Natrum Carb 6C to 30C - A remedy for sunstroke with a headache that feels like a weight on the head. The person may experience weakness and exhaustion and be sensitive to heat. Important Remedy for Sunstroke when the patient is susceptible to changes in temperature. Good for sensitive people who always seem to get headaches from being in the sun. Remedy for debility and exhaustion and headache caused by the sun. Also good for the chronic effects of sun-stroke. Patient may complain of tiredness and extreme weakness due to hot weather. In most cases, the complaints may get worse with a little exertion.

Gelsemium 6C to 30C - Useful for sunstroke with dizziness, heavy eyelids and a headache that starts at the back of the head and radiates forward. The person may feel weak and lethargic and experience trembling. Light headed, droopy, drowsy, thirstless despite the heat. Occasional chills running up and down the spine. Useful in sun-stroke where there is a high temperature with drowsiness and they may feel weak and lethargic and experience trembling, tendency to coma.

Lachesis 6C to 30C - A good remedy for sun-headaches or after being in the sun where there is faintness and dizziness. The key indicator is the person feels worse after a sleep or nap.

Sun (heat) Stroke

Belladonna 6C to 30C - Indicated for sudden, intense symptoms of sunstroke, including high fever, throbbing headache, red face and dilated pupils. The person may be restless, delirious and sensitive to light and noise. Skin is flushed, hot and dry, rapid strong pulse, pupils are fixed and dilated. Headache that is better for dark, silence and rest. The headache can have violent shooting pains in the head which come and go suddenly making the patient cry out. Heat about the head with cold feet. Blood shot eyes and visible throbbing of the carotids. Use for Sunstroke with Congestion of the Head and Face. People needing Belladonna will experience a burning sensation on the face, a severe congestive headache and redness in the eyes. The patient may faint due to weakness. The skin feels hot, red, and dry, and the complaints may aggravate with the least movement.

Gelsemium 6C to 30C - Light headed, droopy, drowsy, thirstless despite the heat. Occasional chills running up and down the spine. Useful in sun-stroke where there is a high temperature with drowsiness or tendency to coma. In Sunstroke when patient feels dull and drowsy. In such cases, there is weakness along with trembling. The patient may feel dizzy and confused. Works well when there is vertigo with a blurring of vision. In most cases, the patient may feel better on lying down.

Glonoine 6C to 30C - Suitable for sunstroke with a severe headache, pulsating or bursting sensation in the head and a feeling of heat in the head. The person may have a flushed face, dilated pupils and experience dizziness or confusion. Throbbing, bursting headache with a hot face and sweaty skin. A great remedy for the effects of sunstroke and congestive headaches. Indicated when the patient has a severe, sudden headache with a throbbing sensation. The patient complains of heaviness in the head, and a feeling that the head is about to burst. In most cases, the pain in the head may get better after sleeping.

Lachesis 6C to 30C - Good remedy for sun-headaches or after being in the sun where there is faintness and dizziness. The key indicator is the person feels worse after a sleep or nap. Lachesis is an important remedy for a patient who gets a pale face and may even faint during

Sunstroke. Nausea and vomiting, along with a cutting and pressing headache, may also occur. The head is very sensitive to touch, and the headache may get worse with a change in weather.

Other Remedies to Consider

Bryonia 6C to 30C - Severe Headache worse for even a slight movement. Remedy to think of when the person has an *intense unquenchable thirst for water*. The person is definitely better for lying completely still and quiet.

Cuprum Met 6C to 30C - First remedy to think of for heat exhaustion if the main symptom is *cramping or the person makes jerking motions of the muscles*. There may also be light-headedness, a rapid pulse and a cold sweat.

Lycopodium 6C to 30C - Heat exhaustion with gastric symptoms - flatulence or a heavy stomach immediately after eating and worse 4 - 8pm. They are generally better for uncovering and getting cooled down.

Natrum Mur 6C to 30C - Good for sunstroke with heat in the head and a red face, nausea and vomiting. A bursting headache or pain like 'tiny hammers' banging. There may be fiery zigzags before the eyes. Very thirsty and a marked desire or aversion to salty food.

BELOW FOR YOUR INTEREST IS THE OPINION OF A MASTER HOMOEOPATH. NOTE ACONITUM THE ONE THAT I AND A LOT OF OTHERS MISSED OUT, THAT'S WHY HE IS A MASTER. THIS IS REPEATED IN THE CATTLE SECTION.

Heat Prostration for Cattle

George MacLeod (McLeod) (1912 – 1995) MRCVS DVSM Veterinary FF. Hom

Sunstroke

Direct rays of the sun on the head may produce dilation of cerebral blood-vessels which in severe cases can cause paralysis. **Symptoms** - Excitement and restlessness are quickly evident and in the less acute case paralysis of certain muscles takes place, finally leading to failure of the respiratory centre.

Homoeopathic Treatment

Aconitum Napellus 12X. This remedy given at once will help calm the animal and reduce excitement. Dose - one every half-hour for four doses.

Beladonna 1M. A most useful remedy for cerebral congestion. Generally there may be visible throbbing of surface vessels, with excitement and dilated pupils. Dose - One every half-hour for four doses. It should be alternated with Aconitum.

Glonoine 30C. One of the main remedies for exposure to sun. The animal exhibits signs of pain in the head, such as throwing the head against any convenient object or banging on the ground. Recumbency is usual with unsteadiness of movement if made to rise. This remedy will do much to reduce the tension in the cerebral blood vessels. Dose - one every hour for four doses.

Heat Exhaustion

Accumulation of body heat may arise after exposure to a long spell of hot weather when the heat builds up in the body. It can be made worse by exercise. Factors which may influence this condition apart from heat are lack of proper oxygenation, fatigue, and insufficient intake of water, together with unnecessary handling, during prolonged hot weather. **Symptoms -** Rapid respirations are a constant sign along with depression and anorexia. The mouth is usually open and frothy mucus accumulates. A rapid pulse is present, while an extremely high temperature is constant. The conjunctivae become congested and motor reflexes are lost.

Homoeopathic Treatment

Glonoine 30C. As Glonoine 30C for Sunstroke.

Natrum Muriaticum 30C. A useful remedy for stabilising the salt metabolism and preventing loss. Dose: one every three hours for four doses.

Sulphur 30C. This remedy is useful for reducing the effects of heat generally, enabling the animal to make a quicker recovery. Dose - one dose every two hours for four

doses. The administration of these remedies will help the action of cold water applications, which are always extremely valuable in reducing heat.

Pigs and Heat Stress

Pigs are going to have a problem with climate change as they are unable to cool themselves with perspiration as humans can do, which makes them very susceptible to heat stress. Another problem is that they also get sunburnt, and should not be exposed to long periods of direct sunlight or extremes of temperature. Problems may begin at about 25 Celsius. Outdoor pigs survive the heat naturally by finding shady cool areas with a breeze and increasing water uptake along with lying on a cool surface. As the heat rises they would then start looking for places where they could make or find some where to make a mud bath, or head off to their local mud bath and have a roll in the mud to cool down with the mud also being their sun tan lotion. Pigs that are being fattened especially in summer can suffer heat stress from about 20 Celsius onwards, remember calories make heat. Signs of heat exhaustion in pigs can include open mouth breathing, panting and making more noise than usual, blotchy skin, stiffness, muscle tremors, and a reluctance to move. They will also reduce the amount of food they are consuming to slow the internal heat that is produced by digestion. When the animal starts panting very hard, that's when you are in trouble, especially if the heats going to last for a long time. A good start would be soaking a big towel with cold water and putting it on the pig's neck and back along with a long cool drink. Always check the young first as they are usually the ones that are affected first and the most, especially if mum stops producing milk, followed by the sows as they have a higher death rate during heat stress. Continuous access to clean water is critical for pig health. The key clinical signs and symptoms include a high respiratory rate, distress and a rectal temperature of 43°C. Part of the problem with pigs is that they don't sweat and they have small lungs so panting may not give much relief.

Symptoms of Heat Stress

Respiration increases and may lead to panting.
Lethargic when moving, slowed down.
Feed intake is slowed so as to reduce internal heat.
Reduced growth in feeder pigs and maybe the young.
Reduced milk production in lactating sows.
General loss in weight.
Diarrhoea.
Increased water consumption.
Increased urine output.
Muscle trembling and weakness.

Transporting Pigs during Hot Days

Hots days are not good for transporting pigs especially when it gets over 25 Celsius. It is best to avoid transporting pigs on hot or humid days. If you have to move them ensure they are transported in a covered and well ventilated trailer to avoid sunburn and to have a cooling breeze. The hotter it gets the more you have to reduce the loading density for example above 25C reduce loading by 10 percent and the hotter it gets consider more so as to allow the pigs to lie on the floor and ensure they are having a good breeze pass through them. On arrival unloaded immediately and give access to cool clean water and shade.

Cattle and Heat Stress

As some places are more affected by climate change then others along with the related water changes due to the changing weather patterns, there will be many changes in the breeds of cattle as their suitability in certain areas becomes questioned. A lot of the British breeds are not going to like the heat and no doubt there will be a lot of experimenting with crossbreeds now and into the near future. Cattle are more prone to heat stress than sheep and goats. Beef cattle with black hair suffer more from direct solar radiation than those with lighter hair, while those with pink skin are at risk of sunburn. Lactating cattle are more susceptible than dry cows because of the additional metabolic heat generated during lactation while high producing dairy cows are more affected by extreme heat than lower producing cows. Heavy cattle over 450kg are more susceptible than lighter ones to sun and heat stroke and no doubt all the overweight ones are.

Symptoms of Heat Stress

Reduced feed intake or change in feeding.
Cattle stand rather than lie down.
Bunching up in shaded areas.
Bunching up around the water trough.
Rapid shallow breathing or open mouth breathing.
Respiration rate increase with the heat.
Panting at higher temperatures.
Increased saliva production.
Lack of coordination and trembling.
Heatwaves can cause rapid dehydration in calves.
Sick or stressed cattle do not like heatwaves.

In regards to heat, cattle and cows do not sweat effectively and rely on respiration to cool themselves. To add to the burden the fermentation process within the rumen creates additional heat which accumulates during the day and dissipates at night when it is cooler. This creates a problem during heatwaves, especially if they last a long time and even worse when the temperatures just keep on going up. Cattles core temperature peaks 2 hours after the peak temperature of the day and then it takes at least 6 hours for their heat load to dissipate. Heavy cattle have a harder time with heat stress due to increased fat deposition and will need more time for recovery. As respiration is used for cooling keep your eyes open for animal's with respiratory problems as they will fare worse and like the canary in the cage they should give you the first warnings of what may come if the temperatures do not drop. Water is the fastest and quickest way for cattle to reduce their core body temperature so you have to ensure that they are able to get it which creates more problems. As we know that the climate is only going to get worse it should now be a priority to add more water troughs and more shady cool areas for stock and allow them the time they need to get used to the changes.

Heat Prostration for Cattle

George MacLeod (McLeod) (1912 – 1995) MRCVS DVSM Veterinary FF. Hom

Sunstroke

Direct rays of the sun on the head may produce dilation of cerebral blood-vessels which in severe cases can cause paralysis. **Symptoms** - Excitement and restlessness are quickly evident and in the less acute case paralysis of certain muscles takes place, finally leading to failure of the respiratory centre.

Homoeopathic Treatment

Aconitum Napellus 12X. This remedy given at once will help calm the animal and reduce excitement. Dose - one every half-hour for four doses.

Beladonna 1M. A most useful remedy for cerebral congestion. Generally there may be visible throbbing of surface vessels, with excitement and dilated pupils. Dose - One every half-hour for four doses. It should be alternated with Aconitum.

Glonoine 30C. One of the main remedies for exposure to sun. The animal exhibits signs of pain in the head, such as throwing the head against any convenient object or banging on the ground. Recumbency is usual with unsteadiness of movement if made to rise. This remedy will do much to reduce the tension in the cerebral blood vessels. Dose - one every hour for four doses.

Heat Exhaustion

Accumulation of body heat may arise after exposure to a long spell of hot weather when the heat builds up in the body. It can be made worse by exercise. Factors which may influence this condition apart from heat are lack of proper oxygenation, fatigue, and insufficient intake of water, together with unnecessary handling, during prolonged hot weather. **Symptoms -** Rapid respirations are a constant sign along with depression and anorexia. The mouth is usually open and frothy mucus accumulates. A rapid pulse is present, while an extremely high temperature is constant. The conjunctivae become congested and motor reflexes are lost.

Homoeopathic Treatment

Glonoine 30C. As Glonoine 30C for Sunstroke.

Natrum Muriaticum 30C. A useful remedy for stabilising the salt metabolism and preventing loss. Dose: one every three hours for four doses.

Sulphur 30C. This remedy is useful for reducing the effects of heat generally, enabling the animal to make a quicker recovery. Dose - one dose every two hours for four doses. The administration of these remedies will help the action of cold water applications, which are always extremely valuable in reducing heat.

Horses and Heat Stress

The best example we can use for Heat Stress is the racing horse. Exercise results in the generation of heat, and in a horse race the horses can produce enough heat to increase the body temperature by one degree Celsius for every minute of the race. For your average non-working horse its problems in climate change could be high temperatures and humidity, lack of wind or air movement in housing along with heat, poor ventilation and dehydration, while outside there would be exposure to direct sunlight and heat with maybe hot dry winds and not much shade. A horse's natural response to heat is usually to increase their sweating along with the rate of breathing and to move more blood into the capillaries under the skin so as to cool it a bit before entering the main blood stream again, that is of course if it didn't have a cold drink of water first.

Symptoms of Heat Stress

Excessive or profuse sweating.

No sweating. (Runout of spare water).

Skin that is dry and hot.

Reduced feed intake.

Rapid shallow breathing or panting.

Flared nostrils.

Unpredictable behaviour and gait.

Very high body temperature.

High respiratory rate.

High heart rate – over 50 beats per minute.

High rectal temperature over 39 degrees Celsius.

A simple test to determine if the horse is dehydrated is to pinch the horse's skin on the neck and see if it resumes its original position immediately, if it takes a while to resume its normal position then it's dehydrated. As usual it is the old and young that can get into difficulties fairly fast so always keep an eye on them when it gets too hot. The very young and foals have a very poor heat regulating ability and can overheat just by standing in the sun so great care is needed for them especially if mum isn't all that bright. It is very worthwhile to have handy a large salt and electrolyte formula that you could use in emergencies, which should be easily found at any good horse shop. Horses that are overweight and not used regularly, along with not being used to hard work are some of the main victims of heat stroke. Horses with difficulty in breathing and looking stressed that develop diarrhoea or signs of colic, or stop sweating are in need of help. Take the horse to a cool and shady area and hose down the horse gently, if you fear the water is to cold sponge the horse down or do a mixture of both. As the horse settles direct the hose to the insides of the legs, head and neck areas following the areas where there are large blood vessels so as to help cool the blood, which in turn will help cool the body internally. Don't forget the wet towel trick especially for the young. Excess water must be scraped off afterwards unless there is a good breeze, as water in the coat on a hot, humid, still day will act as an insulator and it will quickly warm up again. You can use fans to cool and help evaporate the water which will increase the cooling. Offer a bit of water along with water dosed with electrolytes and let them choose which they want but slow them down if they get to greedy. Sometimes it can take an hour or more to get the temperature back to normal. Allow the horse to recover for about 10 days keeping a good eye on them. Restrict exercising your horse to the early morning and the cool of the evening when it is the coolest. If they liked and chose the Electrolytes before you can also add it to their feed regime for a few days to replace essential salts lost through sweating.

Sheep and Heat Stress

Heat stress in sheep is a significant concern, more so in climate change where weather becomes unpredictable, unreliable and extremes become normal. Here the cold breeds will be affected the most as they tend to have shorter bodies and legs, short thick ears and denser fleeces, so these will have a very real risk of fatalities if signs are not recognised early and steps taken to reduce the risks. High temperatures will also affect feed intake, growth rates, fertility, conception rates and are often accompanied by high humidity which makes the situation worse. The hotter the summers get the more the fodder will be affected and to make it worse the rain may change its normal patterns and what may have been good pastures will turn not so good, maybe now is a good time for a rethink and a change in plans. As you know, plenty of fresh cool water is needed to keep sheep healthy and heat stress free, so now is the time to increase the number of troughs and shade so you are prepared for the worst, and save yourself from the problem of all the troughs being over crowed and causing problems. On average sheep will drink one to two gallons (3.7 litres to 7.4) of water a day, with lactating females needing more. Young animals need to drink more often as they have a faster metabolism but only a small tummy.

Symptoms of Heat Stress

Shade seeking.

Crowding at water troughs.

Bunching to seek shade from other sheep.

1/. Open mouth breathing or panting.

2/. Head extended, tongue protruding, profuse salivation.

1 is the beginning, 2 is really bad.

Increased Respiration.

Increased Respiration with deep flank movements.

Wetting head in a water trough.

Weakness or inability to stand.

Rectal temperature above 41°C. (urgent)

Front legs held in a wide stance.

In extreme heat sheep will decrease their grazing time and spend more time in the shade, especially during the heat of the day, and will graze mostly in the evening and early morning hours. If you find heat-stressed animals move them to a cool, shaded area with good air circulation and for those that are in serious trouble with their head extended and tongue protruding it's time to start to lower body temperature. Sheep should be cooled by applying rubbing alcohol to the area between their rear legs as this area is not covered with wool and has a lot of vascular activity which means we will be cooling not only the skin but the blood as well, as it travels back to the heart. Don't accidently set the poor thing on fire by smoking or having it next to an electric fence. For sheep we do not wet the wool areas as this will actually make matters worse as air will not be able to pass through the fleece. With a hose carefully wet the underside and legs avoiding wool areas along with trying to get a breeze flowing in the same area. Work slowly but surely as you do not want to give a stressed animal the shock of a rapid change as that may be the end especially for the old and young. Other cooling treatments include ice applications and cool water enemas, but only do those for the first time with a vet who can show you how to do it properly and what to do if something goes wrong. Always offer heat-stressed sheep ample water and encourage them to drink small amounts and observe how they are handling it. If you have a water misting bottle it makes it easier to cool the legs and belly and any other place where there is no wool.

Goats and Heat Stress

Goats are similar to sheep in heat stress especially the Angora Goats which like sheep have fleece and the problems that go with it, but have an advantage by having horns which can act like a cooling radiator in a car due to the amount of blood supply flowing through the horns. A cold pack wrapped around the horns may help with cooling but not a frozen one as we don't want give them a brain freeze. Other than the Angora, most goats handle the heat far better and a lot of them are breed for the heat such as the Anglo - Nubians who I helped farm in the tropics with their long floppy ears which help in cooling and long legs which keep them high from the grounds radiating heat. Lactating goats require more water in order to produce milk. As usual the very young and the very old goat will be less heat-tolerant, while the darker coloured goats attract more of the sun's heat and can overheat faster than a white goat. Sunburn can be a problem with light-skinned and coloured goats. Heat stress can lead to heat exhaustion or heat stroke. Providing shade and plenty of fresh water help most goat varieties avoid heat stress.

Symptoms of Heat Stress

Shade seeking.

Crowding at water troughs.

Bunching to seek shade.

Open mouth breathing or panting.

The goats become lethargic.

Increased Respiration Rate.

Weakness or inability to stand.

Rectal temperature above 40°C. (urgent)

Similar to Sheep, Goats pant a lot when the weather is hot. If a goat can't stop panting, stops eating and drinking, and can't get up, it is most likely suffering from heat stress. Rectal temperatures over 40 degrees Celsius are a serious threat and cooling will need to be done along with shade, water and a cool area to recover. Non wool goats can be cooled down using water misting bottles or a fine mist hose especially on long floppy ears (be careful not to get water in the ears) and the horns which can act as cooling radiators along with spraying the rest of the body. If the air is not moving then bring out a few fans. Give the Goat access to cool clean water, small amounts regularly. The main method of transferring heat from a goat varies based upon the air temperature and **humidity,** which is the main killer in the equation. Evaporation will remove heat from the goat but it is critical that the humidity not be very high. Evaporation rates are increased when air passing above the coat has a lower humidity.

Dogs and Working Dogs Heat Stress

Dogs don't sweat as humans do instead they release heat by panting and sweating through their paw pads and nose. If they cannot cool themselves their temperature begins to rise. Be aware of how hard your dog is working in the heat, especially when there is High Humidity. If the heat and humidity are high save the work for another day if you can, and always plan your work with the help of the weather forecast. If they must work, it should only be during the cool times of the day, and they must have regular breaks with access to water and shade. Carry water with you if possible and offer small amounts often. Stop work for a dog suspected of suffering from heat stress and check them out and offer water, if you are still worried put them in a water trough and cover their back with water and see how they react. If you are still not happy put them in the shade with a cool breeze if you can.

Symptoms of Heat Stress

Heat stress – Increased thirst and panting

Dry nose (caused by dehydration)

Heat Exhaustion - Heavy Panting and Weakness

Heat Stroke – Drooling, Dizziness, Collapse.

Increased heart rate and breathing

May be vomiting and diarrhoea.

Muscle tremors and seizures.

Collapse.

Ensure your working dogs have access to shade and a source of clear fresh water at all times when they are kennelled or resting. Ice cubes in a dog's water bowl will help to keep water cool. Do not leave dogs tied up on the back of a ute in the sun and on days over 28C dogs must have a layer of insulating material between them and the metal tray. Always park in the shade and provide water and breeze if you can. Do not leave dogs locked in parked cars. Begin treatment for Heatstroke by moving the dog to a cool shaded area, hopefully with a breeze and begin cooling your dog by wetting down their body with a hose or bucket, but avoid the face. I used to start at the back using my hand to push the fur upward and a low pressure hose following and then do the sides. If there is no breeze then get a fan out to make one as we need the evaporation of the water to do the cooling. Keep doing this for a while and they will generally let you know when feeling better. For pets leave them at home during heatwaves as much as possible with plenty of water and shade and do not force the animal to exercise in hot, humid weather. Exercise pets in the cool of the early morning or evening so as to prevent foot burns from the tar on the roads and hot concrete. Because a dog is much closer to the ground hot asphalt and concrete can heat up quickly, and its paws can sustain burns or injuries. Dogs can get sunburned so protect hairless and light-coated dogs with sunscreen when they will be outside in the sun for an extended period of time. Put sunscreen or zinc on exposed areas of pink skin. Animals with long coats can be clipped to increase comfort in hot weather.

Cats and Heat Stress

Heat exhaustion is the prelude to heatstroke, so you have to move fast before the condition deteriorates. Signs to look out for in Cats are restlessness and restless behaviour as they try to find a cool place, which is usually under the house lying on the cool soil and if they are lucky a nice breeze. Other signs are panting, excessive grooming, drooling, pacing up and down and sweaty paws which are all an effort to cool down. Heatstroke occurs in Cats at about 40 degrees Celsius

Symptoms of Heat Stress
Panting or trouble breathing.
Panting increases.
Drooling, restlessness.
Diarrhoea.
Vomiting.
Staggering, Lethargy.
Muscle tremors, Seizures.
Increased Heart rate.
Disorientation.
Red flushed tongue or gums.
Little to no urine, Coma.

Cats that are at high risk of heat stroke are the old and young, those with a health problem, the fat cat and the flat faced breeds such as Persian or Burmese. Cats with long thick coats need to be trimmed before the heat of summer begins. Prevention is the best way to go especially if you know a heatwave is coming, find the coolest area in the house and set the cat up there with plenty of cool water. That should hopefully save them from burning their feet on hot concrete or tar or dehydrating in the hot breeze. Also on the worst hot days consider giving them wet cat food but in smaller amounts spread out during the day as this would take a lot of workload off the digestive system and keep up the hydration. Our old cat that was fairly bright always went under the house in hot weather and cooled herself on the nice cool soil. If you think your cat is suffering from heat stress take them inside to a cool room and have a feel of the floor temperature to see if it is cool. In severe cases where you know the cat is in trouble start with a temperature check which is done rectally with the normal temperature being just slightly over 38 degrees Celsius to 39.2. Temperatures over and above 40 degrees Celsius are a cause of alarm. Provide cool water and encourage them to drink, but not too much at a time. If the cat has had a drink but still looks bad then we have to cool them manually. Find a water bottle that can be used as a mister for spraying and gently and slowly spray the tummy and chest and get a fan set on low speed breezing into the tummy and chest area. If they are not complaining but seem to need more help you can get 2 hand towels and soak them in water and ring them out but not too much, then scruff the towels up and put the first one between the front paws and then point the fan at it but not too close and see what happens. What we are doing is using the evaporation to cool down the cat. If the cat is happy do the same with the rear legs and aim the fan at the middle of the cat. Adding a small amount of rubbing alcohol to the water can also help speed up the evaporation and cooling effect. Check the temperature every 10 minutes so you know what is happening.

Poultry Heat Stress - Chickens

Here we will only deal with chickens as they are the most common small acreage and home reared poultry and are similar to turkeys in heat stress. Ducks and Geese will just take over the swimming pool in a heat wave and probably be happy in a bath tub under a shady tree. Chickens that are too hot will pant and spread their wings to release body heat. Panting releases water into the air which evaporates and helps to cool the chicken, but you can only do that for so long as eventually it will cause dehydration and a pH imbalance. High humidity decreases heat loss from the lungs which makes the birds more prone to heat stress. When the temperature starts to get to hot for chickens they naturally lose heat through their comb, wattles and other areas not covered by feathers and no doubt by a long cool drink. Poultry should not be wet down unless there is a breeze to aid the cooling process and increase air movement around them. This can be done with fans, ventilation, or wind movement. Warm water is less effective for cooling chickens and will cause fungi, mould, bacteria, and other microbes to grow in water which create other problems. You can also add electrolyte solutions to the drinking water in heat waves so as to help prolong the time till dehydration becomes a problem but only do this for no more than 3 days.

Symptoms of Heat Stress

Panting.

Spreading Wings.

Increased thirst.

Lethargy – slowed down.

Decrease in egg laying.

Chickens do not have sweat glands so one of the main ways they try to cool down is by spreading their wings especially when there is a breeze around. If you see them doing this then it's time to get the fan out. Heat stress can cause a decrease in eggs as mentioned before but also dehydration which decreases the water in the egg and electrolytes in the body. Layers can also become calcium deficient which will cause the egg shells to become thinner and weaker. Chickens in heat can also lose weight and become susceptible to other diseases. A good rule of thumb is that when temperatures rise between 24 to 27 degrees C, it is time to check and begin cooling off your chickens. If temperatures are closer to 37 degrees or beyond, it can be dangerous. Always plan for the worst and hope for the best. During a heat wave feed chickens during the early morning or evening, the coolest parts of the day. Remember calories are a measure of heat, food actually makes you hotter. Keeping the coop cool is an excellent way to make sure your flock stays comfortable during hot weather. Regularly clean out litter as a build-up of litter that has started to decay produces heat, so by removing litter you lower the moisture in the coop, which reduces the relative humidity. Make sure your coop has grass around it and not bare dirt as grass absorbs heat, while dirt reflects heat. Always place a coop where there is a breeze as this is the best way to lower heat and keep up the ventilation. Keeping the water where the breeze exits the coops can help in reducing the humidity inside the coops. Air flow removes hot air and humidity. If you cannot get sufficient natural airflow install fans.

Making your Own Fire Trailer

Here we will go back to the beginning. I saw my first Fire Trailer in use in 2006 on a farm I was living on in South Australia 50Ks north of Adelaide City. As it was very hot there was a fire ban. The area around Adelaide is very rocky which makes it very annoying for the farmers. In the early 18th century convicts starting working on the problem by clearing the fields of rocks and using the rocks to fence the paddocks. It was a good idea at the time but in the future it created a problem for tractors using slashers to keep the grass down as the paddocks were littered with small rocks which cause big sparks when the blades hit them which in turn starts fires that can get out of control fast especially if the wind picks up which seems to happen every time you hit a rock. In times of fire danger when you had to use the slasher you would hook up the fire trailer and park it in the middle of the paddock that you were slashing. The fire trailer was mostly made up of bits and pieces found around the farm and put together. The main bed for the equipment was an old 4x6 foot common trailer which had been strengthened on the floor so as to support the 1000 litre IBC tank and light chains each side with large fence strainers to tension the tank to the trailer. The wheels had 4wd tyres that were wider and stronger along with all the wheel bearings being renewed. This trailer had the petrol engine water pump at the front, mounted on the A frame of the trailer with the pump facing the trailer and the pump motor facing the vehicle. The main hose attached to the pump was the red standard fire hose that you would usually see on the walls of government buildings looking like a red circle on the wall with the black thin hose (Red Fire Hose Reel) which you can usually get very cheaply at the local auctions. Some people like the pump and hose at the front of the trailer while other like it at the back of the trailer. The 1000 litre IBC tank is 4 x 4 feet so on a 4 x 6 Trailer you have 2 feet at the back to mount the pump and the hose wheel. Make the mounting for the hose reel very strong so someone standing on the back can support themselves and use a hose at the same time as this is how they commonly put out the reoccurring spot fires with the driver heading to the fires and the person at the back putting them out. The design for your fire trailer is only limited by your imagination and must be set up by you for your own conditions and needs. You could do this as a joint project with your neighbours or other farmers in the area which could save you a lot of money with an example being buying your pump and other equipment in bulk for a discount which has another advantage of many people using the same equipment so they are familiar with it which is very helpful in emergencies. If you have a group networking together you could have a base station that could invest in a few drones that will give you the advantage of where the fires are in your area or when to run away. It's up to your imagination or for some just survival as this has been well and truly proved now and has saved many life's in Australia especially in the hills and ranges where the roads are easily blocked and the only ones that can save you are you and your neighbours. Don't forget fire trailers can also be used for lots of other purposes such as filling up long distance water troughs, mobile cleaning units, mobile cooling units for heat stressed animals or whatever your imagination come up with. We will end by showing you a cheap and basic modern unit designed solely for firefighting.

BASIC - Pull Start - Fire Fighter 1000L Trailer
A$2,241.00

Locally made Australian Galvanised Chassis

1350Kg Axles, Running Gear

Pull start 6.5hp generic engine (Remanufactured)

Up to 60m head (pumping vertically up)

Up to 8m suction (sucking vertically up)

Up to 200 Liters Per Minute

Reconditioned Firex Red Fire Hose Reel

36 Meter 19mm hose with brass twist nozzle

B-Grade Reconditioned IBC 1000 L Tank

Reconditioned Rims and Tyres

Economy clamp on Jockey Wheel

Mudguards

Fittings
https://egritech.square.site

www.ingramcontent.com/pod-product-compliance
Lightning Source LLC
Chambersburg PA
CBHW081106290526
45795CB00006B/2024